A Concise Guide to
# Borderline Personality Disorder

If I had to suggest a definitive book that clinicians in practice need to be more immediately helpful to patients who have borderline personality disorder (BPD), it's Paris's *A Concise Guide to Borderline Personality Disorder.* An alternative to a technically focused manualized therapy, this book offers an integrated synthesis of the current state of knowledge about BPD written by an expert in the field who understands what the typical clinician who won't practice a specialized approach needs in order to be informed about this complex disorder.

—**Lois W. Choi-Kain, MD, MEd,** Director, Gunderson Personality Disorders Institute, Belmont, MA; Associate Professor of Psychiatry, Harvard Medical School, Boston, MA, United States; Distinguished Fellow, American Psychiatric Association

Dr. Paris is a consummate clinical educator who has influenced generations of mental health clinicians. This book distills a lifetime of clinical wisdom and blends it with Paris's deep knowledge and masterful critical appraisal of the research literature. This practical guide has something for everyone. It is essential reading for trainees and practicing clinicians in all mental health disciplines.

—**Andrew Chanen, MBBS (Hons), BMedSci (Hons), MPM, PhD, FRANZCP,** Professor, Orygen, Parkville, VIC, and The University of Melbourne, Melbourne, VIC, Australia

Practical, research-informed, and clinically focused, Joel Paris has given us an essential guide to BPD diagnosis and treatment. This book is like having an on-hand professional consultant, full of wise, evenly balanced advice and case examples on how to personalize treatment.

—**Brin F. S. Grenyer, PhD,** Professor of Psychology, University of Wollongong, Wollongong, NSW, Australia; Director of the Project Air Strategy for Personality Disorders

This is a deeply instructive text on the treatment of borderline personality disorder. It is not only richly informative but also written in a very straightforward and readily understood manner.

—**Thomas A. Widiger, PhD,** Professor of Psychology, University of Kentucky, Lexington, KY, United States; Editor, *Oxford Handbook of Personality Disorders*

This is a well-organized account of borderline personality disorder that provides a broad and concise overview that should appeal to the targeted readership. The overall approach is balanced and grounded in relevant evidence.

—**John Livesley, MD, PhD, FRSC,** Professor Emeritus, Department of Psychiatry, University of British Columbia, Vancouver, BC, Canada

# JOEL PARIS

A Concise Guide to
# Borderline Personality Disorder

AMERICAN PSYCHOLOGICAL ASSOCIATION

Published by
American Psychological Association
750 First Street, NE
Washington, DC 20002
https://www.apa.org

Order Department
https://www.apa.org/pubs/books
order@apa.org

Typeset in Charter and Interstate by Circle Graphics, Inc., Reisterstown, MD

Printer: Gasch Printing, Odenton, MD
Cover Designer: Anthony Paular Design, Newbury Park, CA

**Library of Congress Cataloging-in-Publication Data**

Names: Paris, Joel, 1940- author.
Title: A concise guide to borderline personality disorder / by Joel Paris.
Description: Washington, DC : American Psychological Association, [2025] |
    Includes bibliographical references and index.
Identifiers: LCCN 2024033602 (print) | LCCN 2024033603 (ebook) | ISBN
    9781433844034 (paperback) | ISBN 9781433844041 (ebook)
Subjects: LCSH: Borderline personality disorder. | Borderline personality
    disorder--Treatment.
Classification: LCC RC569.5.B67 P373 2025 (print) | LCC RC569.5.B67
    (ebook) | DDC 616.85/852--dc23/eng/20241220
LC record available at https://lccn.loc.gov/2024033602
LC ebook record available at https://lccn.loc.gov/2024033603

https://doi.org/10.1037/0000440-000

*Printed in the United States of America*

10 9 8 7 6 5 4 3 2 1

*This book is dedicated to the clinicians and students
who have worked with me in treatment teams
over the last 25 years.*

# Contents

*Acknowledgments*                                                                                    *ix*

**Introduction: Practical Approaches to the Complex Challenges
of Borderline Personality Disorder**                                                                3

**I. RESEARCH**                                                                                      **9**

    1. Diagnosis and Misdiagnosis                                               11
    2. Prevalence, Precursors, and Outcomes                                      33
    3. A Biopsychosocial Theory of Borderline Personality Disorder              47

**II. TREATMENT**                                                                                    **63**

    4. Treatment Methods                                                         65
    5. Access to Therapy for Borderline Personality Disorder                    85
    6. The Problem of Suicidality                                               99
    7. Summary and Future Directions                                            111

*References*                                                                                        *115*
*Index*                                                                                             *139*
*About the Author*                                                                                  *145*

# Acknowledgments

I extend my thanks to APA Publishing, in particular to Susan Reynolds, for suggesting that I write this book, and to Molly Gage, for coordinating the peer review process.

Some sections of Chapter 3 appeared in an earlier form in a journal article (Paris, 2023a).

# A Concise Guide to
# Borderline Personality Disorder

# INTRODUCTION

*Practical Approaches to the Complex Challenges of Borderline Personality Disorder*

Borderline personality disorder (BPD) is a diagnosis that describes patients who are often seen in clinical practice but who are generally considered difficult to treat. The clinical picture of BPD is complex and derives from multiple domains: emotion dysregulation, widespread impulsivity, and highly problematic intimate relationships. Most of these patients seriously consider suicide, and many attempt it. Some (fortunately, a minority) will take their own lives. Thus, BPD is a major challenge for psychotherapists and other mental health clinicians.

However, we now know much more about this disorder: what risk factors are associated with it, how it changes over the life span, and how it is best managed in therapy. This book offers clinicians a practical and evidence-based approach to making a diagnosis in patients who are often misunderstood and misdiagnosed. We also know how to effectively treat most cases of BPD.

BPD has been the subject of many books and thousands of journal articles. This includes a longer book of my own, revised a few years ago in a second edition (Paris, 2020c). However, the present volume will not be a shorter version of that book. Even after 5 years, further research has shed additional light on some crucial clinical issues. Moreover, my own views about BPD have continued to evolve and change. Unlike the longer book, in this volume I will

https://doi.org/10.1037/0000440-001
*A Concise Guide to Borderline Personality Disorder*, by J. Paris

not attempt to summarize and evaluate large bodies of published research. My intent is to provide a practical message for busy therapists who want to understand the big picture. Moreover, it is not necessary to be an expert to understand BPD. For readers who want to dive more deeply into empirical data, throughout the chapters I will refer to key articles and books that summarize a large scientific literature.

With this rationale in mind, I have written this book in a user-friendly style to make it concise and to the point. I will inform readers about what I can conclude after a half-century of work as a clinician and researcher. Most of what I have to say will be based on empirical evidence. Some issues about BPD are still contested and debated, but most of what I will present here can be considered a consensus of evidence-based opinion. Where important problems have not yet benefited from research, I draw on my clinical experience.

This book will also offer a perspective on BPD that is different from the ideas of other experts. As my views have evolved, I am now convinced that understanding this disorder requires the application of a biopsychosocial model. There is a crucial biological background to BPD that reflects the heritable component in this disorder. There are equally crucial psychological components that derive from adverse life experiences (Porter et al., 2020). Finally, there is a social component related to cultural norms and values.

Unfortunately, many of the best-known models of BPD consider only one of these domains (i.e., biological, psychological, social). I will challenge a currently popular model associated with what is being called *complex posttraumatic stress disorder*. This book will show that although childhood trauma is associated with BPD, and worsens its prognosis, it is not the primary cause of the disorder.

The focus of this book will be the development of a model that guides an eclectic and integrated approach to treatment. Thus, BPD need not be seen as mainly rooted in abnormal brain circuitry, or as entirely due to traumatic experiences. Instead, its development is best understood in terms of gene–environment interactions. I will apply a similar model to understanding what makes treatment of BPD successful. Over the past few decades, various methods of psychotherapy designed specifically for BPD have been promoted, but each of these approaches tends to describe only one part of the interventions that work for patients. In this book, I propose an eclectic model that integrates ideas drawn from many sources. I also show how well-planned therapies of several kinds can help patients with BPD.[1] You do not have to take courses or follow a manual to manage these cases.

---

[1]Case examples in this book are fictionalized composites. Identifying characteristics have been changed to protect client confidentiality.

Finally, I will show that many (if not most) patients with BPD do not necessarily need years of therapy but can be helped by briefer interventions that can rapidly set them on a road to recovery—often within months rather than years. Moreover, time-limited therapy allows more patients to enter the mental health system and receive treatment that is more specific to the complexity of BPD.

## UNDERSTANDING AND MISUNDERSTANDING BPD

BPD describes a common form of psychopathology that can be diagnosed in nearly 10% of all outpatients with personality disorders (Zimmerman et al., 2005), yet this disorder remains one of the most misunderstood conditions in psychiatry and clinical psychology.

First, consider that the name "borderline" is rather misleading. Although once thought to fall between psychosis and neurosis, the condition lies not on one border but on many. BPD is a very complex diagnosis, presenting with a toxic mix of unstable mood, impulsivity, and unstable relationships.

Many have thought the name of BPD should be changed, that it might more accurately be labeled "emotion regulation disorder," or "emotionally unstable personality disorder." The reason is that dysregulated emotions are a primary feature of BPD. However, they do not tell the whole story. Patients with BPD also experience widespread impulsivity (in particular, chronic suicidality and self-harm) as well as other impulsive features, such as substance use, and eating disorders. The clinical picture is also marked by highly unstable interpersonal relationships that many see as a hallmark of the condition. One cannot diagnose BPD if emotion dysregulation is the only clinical feature.

These intersections between pathological domains lead to another diagnostic problem. BPD has a wide range of symptoms that overlap with other mental disorders. These comorbidities lead to a good deal of misdiagnoses that promote mistreatment. For example, most BPD patients have chronic depression, anxiety, or both, leading them to be treated, sometimes for years, with antidepressants, but these pharmacological agents have little benefit in this population. Moreover, standard cognitive behavior therapy methods have limited efficacy in BPD. This is why most specialists see these patients after other attempts at treatment have failed.

A second difficulty is that many models of the etiology of and treatment for BPD have a weak grounding in evidence. Thus, BPD is often misunderstood as mainly the result of childhood adversities, in particular highly traumatic events. In this model, BPD tends to overlap with diagnoses of posttraumatic stress disorder or complex posttraumatic stress disorder. It is true that many BPD patients (at least one-third) have histories of early trauma, but the majority describe a more subtle risk factor: neglect of their emotions and having those emotions misunderstood, invalidated, or dismissed (Linehan, 1993).

Even if traumatic events are not the primary or the only cause of BPD, they make the course of the disorder more problematic. The majority of patients with BPD do not have a history of childhood trauma (unless you define "trauma" so broadly that it describes any kind of dysfunctional family or problematic relationship). Moreover, only a minority of children who are seriously traumatized grow up to develop BPD. Instead, as hypothesized decades ago by Linehan (1993), most patients struggle with two "hits"—that is, two interacting risk factors—that create a vicious cycle. The first consists of heritable traits that make emotions stronger and more problematic (Amad et al., 2014). The second consists of experiences of having emotions invalidated by family members and caretakers.

The evidence shows that emotional neglect, not trauma, is the most universal psychological risk factor for BPD (Porter et al., 2020). Moreover, life adversity is the "second hit" that amplifies emotions and makes them dysregulated. BPD is unlikely to develop in the absence of heritable traits that lead to high levels of emotionality.

This overemphasis on childhood trauma has led to serious mistakes in planning treatment, with some therapists focusing mainly on early memories. However, that approach fails to understand the complex etiology of BPD, and it fails to help patients cope with a problematic temperament. Most important, it fails to take into account current life problems that can be triggered by a perception that one's emotions are invalidated by other people.

An even more important missing link is the genetics of traits that are heritable risk factors for the disorder. Twin studies (Bornovalova et al., 2009; Skaug et al., 2022) have shown that these factors account for about half the variance in BPD as an outcome. Of course, genes alone do not explain why patients develop BPD, but the disorder is most likely to arise from gene–environment interactions. That means that people who have specific genetic predispositions respond differently and more intensely to adverse life events than those who do not. One cannot understand trauma without taking into consideration the traits that influence the way a person processes life events.

An emphasis on the past has fed the perception that BPD is intractable to treatment. That point of view is, to put matters plainly, wrong. We now know that most patients get better with time and that most specialized treatments are effective. Unfortunately, clinicians tend to be impressed by the minority who keep coming back when the disorder fails to remit. We now have much better and more specific forms of therapy to offer patients with BPD. Successful therapy can damp down emotion dysregulation, bring impulsivity under control, and teach patients the skills they need to manage intimate relationships.

There are now several forms of psychotherapy with demonstrable efficacy and effectiveness for BPD. Unfortunately, as is the case in general for talk therapy, clinicians tend to become attached to one particular method that claims to be superior to its competitors. My view makes use of concepts derived from dialectical behavior therapy (Linehan, 1993) that are combined with ideas from other methods, including good psychiatric management (Sonley & Choi-Kain, 2021), integrated modular treatment (Livesley, 2017), and mentalization-based treatment (Bateman & Fonagy, 2004). Concentration on a single model can prevent clinicians from making their own synthesis of the best ideas from all sources. In this book, I will show that several methods have good research support and that no single approach is necessarily better than any other.

Before applying any of these methods, one has to recognize the disorder. Unfortunately, many clinicians have biases that lead to a failure to make an early diagnosis of BPD. Because of its association with mood swings, BPD can be confused with bipolar disorder. Because most of these patients are chronically depressed, it may be treated (usually unsuccessfully) with antidepressants. Because BPD has multiple comorbidities, it can also be confused with posttraumatic stress disorder or attention-deficit/hyperactivity disorder.

Once recognized, the road to recovery from BPD is open. Successful therapy can damp down emotion dysregulation, bring impulsivity under control, and teach patients the skills they need to handle intimate relationships. BPD is a disorder with many faces, and clinicians need to assess personality and not just symptoms.

BPD also has a variable course and outcome. It usually begins in adolescence, a time when hormones and developmental challenges trigger symptoms even in relatively typical people. But the disorder typically (but gradually) remits during young adulthood and only rarely meets diagnostic criteria by early middle age. Thus, the vast majority of patients get better with time.

Still another problem derives from the belief that BPD patients need to be treated (at great expense) over many years to get better. Although the recovery process varies in length, once things get on the right trajectory improvement gains momentum. The larger problem concerns accessibility to effective and evidence-based psychotherapy, which many, or most, patients cannot afford.

My recommendations for management will be based on a model in which the best ideas for all current forms of therapy can be used; framed within an application of a stepped care model of treatment, in which most patients are treated briefly; and in which only a subset require longer therapy. I will describe our clinical team's specialized program and explain how it often leads to symptomatic remission and how others have applied similar methods, all supported by empirical data. Moreover, although BPD is common in practice, treatment tends to be too expensive or not readily available. For that reason, brief therapy allows easier access to treatment for more patients.

A final point of misunderstanding concerns whether BPD can or should be diagnosed as early as adolescence. I will review data showing that the early teenage years are usually the stage at which the disorder first appears. That said, there can be a significant delay between the onset of symptoms and contact with the mental health system.

BPD is a common clinical problem that therapists find challenging, largely because of its association with suicidal ideas and behaviors. This book was written for clinicians who see these patients and who are looking for practical management tools. I will not advocate the adoption of still another specific therapy with a three-letter acronym—we have enough of those already. Instead, my approach will be integrative and eclectic, combining ideas from multiple sources. BPD patients have unusual ways of feeling, thinking, and behaving, yet a good deal of what works in therapy is close to common sense.

PART **I** RESEARCH

# 1 DIAGNOSIS AND MISDIAGNOSIS

In this chapter, I review the main features of borderline personality disorder (BPD) and describe how a diagnosis is confirmed using either the *Diagnostic and Statistical Manual of Mental Disorders* (5th ed., text rev.; *DSM-5-TR*; American Psychiatric Association, 2022), the Alternate Model for Personality Disorders (AMPD), or the *International Statistical Classification of Diseases and Related Health Problems* (*ICD-11*; World Health Organization, 2019). I will show how BPD can be distinguished from depression, from bipolar disorder, from psychosis, from attention-deficit/hyperactivity disorder (ADHD), from autism, and from either posttraumatic stress disorder (PTSD) or what has been called complex posttraumatic stress disorder (CPTSD).

## THE KEY FEATURES OF BPD

Diagnosing BPD can be difficult. This is because it is a complex disorder, straddling multiple domains. In addition to emotion dysregulation, widespread impulsivity, and unstable relationships (Leichsenring et al., 2023, 2024), about half of these patients also have micropsychotic symptoms, such as depersonalization, paranoid trends, or transient hallucinations (Cavelti

https://doi.org/10.1037/0000440-002
*A Concise Guide to Borderline Personality Disorder*, by J. Paris

et al., 2021). BPD can be especially difficult to diagnose within the *DSM* system because the latter requires counting criteria, and only patients who display more than half of any given criteria receive a diagnosis. Because BPD can manifest so variably and in a number of different domains, *DSM-5-TR* diagnoses can be challenging.

Another difficulty is that there are now several diagnostic systems, each of which describes BPD a little differently. The *DSM* system is the most widely used, but it has problems in that it focuses on counting criteria, so that patients with only more than half of them get the diagnosis. To make diagnosis more coherent, one could either view BPD as lying on a spectrum (Livesley, 2017) or require more criteria to be present (Zanarini, 2005), but given that these approaches do not necessarily align with the current *DSM* designation, diagnoses remain challenging.

It is the complex mix of symptoms that makes diagnosis more difficult. Although it is tempting to think of BPD as entirely a result of pathology in a single domain, all of the features listed in *DSM-5-TR* are closely related (Dixon-Gordon et al., 2020). When emotions are dysregulated, people do impulsive things to distract themselves. And when both emotions and behaviors are dysregulated, close relationships tend to be problematic.

Moreover, BPD patients often have multiple comorbidities (e.g., substance use, eating disorders, depression, anxiety, PTSD). These additional diagnoses might be better called "co-occurrences," because they need to be considered not as separate categories but as deriving from the central features of the disorder (Shah & Zanarini, 2018). Furthermore, adding additional diagnoses makes it more likely that each co-occurrence will be treated separately, leading to practices for which there is insufficient evidence (see Chapter 4). But some comorbidities do require separate management, most particularly severe substance use (Trull et al., 2018) or severe eating disorders (Zanarini et al., 2010), and these conditions should be diagnosed separately.

The features of BPD patients' multiple comorbidities should be considered not as separate diagnoses but as deriving from the central features of the disorder. It is tempting to see BPD patients as having additional diagnoses, such as depression, bipolarity, or PTSD, but that can be a mistake. A search for comorbidities that are believed to be separately treatable fails to view personality traits as a central feature. It also fails to identify a diagnosis that can benefit from specific forms of psychotherapy. In practice, multiple comorbidities are associated with diagnoses of personality disorders (PDs).

Recognizing that a patient has a PD frames symptoms within a broader diagnostic construct. The overall construct of a PD describes difficulties in relation to self and to others, that is, long-term problems finding an identity and a direction in life, as well as unstable and troubled interpersonal relationships (Krueger et al., 2018). PDs are rooted in pathological traits (problematic levels of negative affectivity, detachment, antagonism, and disinhibition) that psychologists have long measured using the five-factor personality model (FFM; Widiger & Costa, 2013). These features are more important than more nonspecific symptoms, such as depression or anxiety. Moreover, viewing BPD in the context of underlying pathological traits can be the basis for effective treatment. On the other hand, misdiagnosing BPD as a disorder that is assumed to respond to medication or to more standard forms of therapy often leads to ineffective treatment.

CASE EXAMPLE 1.1
## THE TYPICAL PRESENTATION OF BPD

Barbara[1] was a 28-year-old woman working only intermittently and living with a friend. She had a history of depression and anxiety that went back to early adolescence. Since that time, Barbara has suffered from chronic suicidal ideation and recurrent self-harm (cutting). Her emotions were difficult to control, and she has flown into rages with intimate partners that had, on several occasions, led to calls to the police. It would take her hours to days to recover from these episodes. Barbara was easily triggered by any perception of rejection from others. Barbara's relationships usually ended after a few months, leading, on several occasions, to her taking overdoses followed by emergency room (ER) visits or hospitalizations. She also had feelings of inner emptiness, associated with frequent binges on alcohol or food. When in a highly emotional state, Barbara reported hearing voices in her head criticizing her. She has been prescribed four different antidepressant drugs, none of which have removed her overall load of psychological symptoms.

This example describes a patient with all the features of BPD: emotion dysregulation, widespread impulsivity, troubled close relationships, and micropsychosis. Although not all patients will have all these features, clinicians should keep in mind the full clinical picture of the disorder.

## BORDERLINE—BUT ON WHAT BORDER?

As acknowledged in the Introduction, BPD has a misleading name. The term "borderline" derives from a theory that patients with these problems fall somewhere between psychosis and neurosis (Stern, 1938). That is not how we think about BPD today. We could change the name of the disorder, but

---

[1]Case examples in this book are fictionalized composites. Identifying characteristics have been changed to protect client confidentiality.

doing so would not make treatment any less challenging, or remove the stigma attached to it (which mainly derives from its association with suicidality). One could make a reasonable argument for calling this clinical picture "emotion dysregulation disorder," because that is a central feature of the disorder (Linehan, 1993), yet patients who experience emotion dysregulation may lack the other features that define BPD.

Because BPD was first described by psychoanalysts, and it did not have a history in mental health practice, it was ignored for many years by clinicians, who tended to be suspicious of such a diagnosis. Moreover, this disorder has had a reputation for being untreatable. Today, decades of research have demonstrated that BPD is a valid mental disorder, that it has a generally good prognosis, and that it is treatable (Paris, 2020c). Even if we could eventually define it more precisely, it would present the same clinical problems.

Now that several thousand research papers, as well as many books, have been published on BPD, and recovery and effective therapies have been documented, patients with this disorder are being recognized more often. However, unneeded confusion might arise from major changes to its diagnostic criteria. As one expert pointed out (Zimmerman, 2016), changes in nomenclature in psychiatry should be based less on theory and more on data showing that doing so makes treatment more effective.

## BPD IN THE *DSM* SYSTEM

Over the past few decades, the various editions of the *DSM* have dominated the diagnosis of mental disorders in North America. The *DSM* has been used worldwide as a guide to research in psychiatry and clinical psychology, yet BPD was not listed as a mental disorder in its earlier editions: *DSM-I* (American Psychiatric Association, 1952) or *DSM-II* (American Psychiatric Association, 1968). I was a student when these two editions were published, and I had heard little about the BPD diagnosis except for warnings from teachers not to use it. BPD played only a marginal role in the clinical literature, mostly in articles by psychotherapists describing clinical experiences instead of data. Then everything changed, with the paradigm shift associated with the construction of *DSM-III* (American Psychiatric Association, 1980). This version of the manual applied a model that prioritized reliability between different observers and listed sets of observable criteria that could be scored as present or absent.

A seminal article by Gunderson and Singer (1975) was the first to describe a method of diagnosing BPD using a set of observable and potentially reliable criteria. This system became, with some modifications, the basis of the definition in *DSM-III*. A list of eight criteria included the features unstable mood, impulsivity, and conflictual relationships. There have been a few modifications since *DSM-IV* (American Psychiatric Association, 1994) added a ninth criterion of dissociation or paranoid trends, but since then the definitions in *DSM-5* (American Psychiatric Association, 2013) and *DSM-5-TR* have not changed.

The current criteria for a *DSM-5-TR* diagnosis of BPD include multiple domains: affective symptoms (affective instability, anger, emptiness), impulsive symptoms (suicidality and a wide range of impulsivity), and problems with close relationships (unstable and intense), as well as identity problems and micropsychotic phenomena (paranoid or dissociative symptoms). This makes the disorder rather complex. Patients are required to meet five out of nine criteria. But by setting the bar relatively low (just more than half), clinical populations that fit into the category are inevitably heterogeneous, both in symptoms and in severity. (When we understand what causes a disease, such as COVID-19, we can make a diagnosis in spite of variations in clinical presentations, but that is not an option in most mental disorders.)

In recent years, categories of all kinds in psychiatric diagnosis have been criticized as artificial and not based on an understanding of the underlying nature of psychopathology (Krueger et al., 2018). Some trait psychologists have recommended that in the absence of knowledge about the causes of mental disorders, clinicians are better advised to measure psychopathology quantitatively, by scoring patients on multiple quantitative trait dimensions (Hopwood et al., 2018). According to this view, because categories are heterogeneous and overlapping, both in symptomatology and etiology, they may not be the best guide to prescribing evidence-based treatment.

Personality disorders (PDs) in *DSM-5* were considered a test case as to whether a shift from categories to quantitative dimensions would be valid or clinically relevant. At this point, the jury is still out. A new system, in which categories are rooted in trait dimensions, remains in a list of proposals requiring more research. Many of the 10 PD categories still listed in *DSM-5-TR* have little or no research behind them—with the notable exception of BPD and antisocial personality disorder, each of which have stimulated thousands of research papers. Most of the others would not survive serious evidence-based critiques of their validity.

Dimensional systems have long been proposed for the diagnosis of PDs and were originally intended to be applied in *DSM-5*. Dimensions have also been considered as a model for all mental disorders, including a proposal to replace the *DSM* with a diagnostic system based on neuroscience (Cuthbert & Insel, 2013), or with a factor-analysis–based system that uses symptom dimensions called the *Hierarchical Taxonomy of Psychopathology* (HiToP; Kotov et al., 2017).

There has been resistance to a move toward dimensional systems. Clinicians, psychiatrists in particular, are used to categories, which are routinely used in medicine as a whole. The most serious objection is that dimensions have not yet been shown to lead to better treatment (Zimmerman, 2016). Another concern is whether adopting an unfamiliar system for making PD diagnoses, or using one that is overly complex, could create a problem (the tendency to ignore PDs) even worse. Still another is that factor analysis of self-reported symptoms is not based on any theory (in contrast, the classification of species is based on evolution). Thus, similar symptoms do not necessarily describe valid dimensions (or categories). Eventually, with more research, we might be able to develop such a theory, but we do not currently have one (Haeffel et al., 2022).

In the work groups for *DSM-5*, a compromise between categories and dimensions was eventually adopted. The new system, called a *hybrid*, has the advantage of retaining categories while basing them on trait dimensions. It was placed in a section of the *DSM-5-TR* relating to diagnoses that require additional research support, and it is now termed the *Alternative Model for Personality Disorders* (AMPD; Krueger et al., 2018). The AMPD is a model in which categories remain but are ultimately based on lower levels of functioning and on scores that describe personality traits. In the past decade, the proponents of the AMPD have published hundreds of papers on this system, and it could eventually become a part of *DSM-6*.

Using the AMPD, one first determines whether there is sufficient reason to consider that a patient has a PD, by scoring the extent to which psychopathology affects both the patient's self-concept and relationships with other people. Then the specific type of PD is determined by measuring the severity of problematic personality traits.

Algorithms based on trait profiles are used to construct specific categories of disorder—of which there would now be only six instead of 10. (The number was originally five, but a lobby for including narcissistic personality disorder succeeded in adding it to the list.) Thus, to diagnose BPD with the AMPD, clinicians need to describe the general features of a PD and then identify the traits associated with BPD: emotional lability, separation anxiety, anxiousness, hostility, depressivity, risk-taking, and impulsivity (Hopwood et al., 2019).

The current diagnostic system for PDs is outmoded, but there is still doubt as to what should replace it. At this point, the AMPD could be the best alternative. Yet many trait psychologists do not like this system, either, because it retains categories. However, although some clinicians may find its algorithms complicated, if the AMPD were adopted they would learn it and use it in practice, at which point complexity might not be a barrier. Nonetheless, a more rigorous methodology could discourage clinicians from making PD diagnoses on the basis of one or two clinical features that come most easily to mind. For now, the AMPD remains a research measure, at least until it is allowed to move into the main body of the manual and replace categories that have been retained from previous editions.

In North America, the *DSM* manuals have had a strong hold for several decades on the way clinicians see their patients. The categories they describe used to be considered provisional, but they have become reified. For all the criticism the manual has faced, few clinicians seem keen to take up any of the alternatives. Yet *DSM* guidelines must be open to change. Having seen the radical rethink that happened when psychiatry adopted *DSM-III*, we know that major changes can happen—and if they make more theoretical and clinical sense, we should adopt them. A system that has the advantage of yielding both categories and dimensions could well be better than what we have now.

This is why I would, in spite of some doubts, be sympathetic to adoption of the AMPD, which combines the advantages of a dimensional approach with the identification of clinically meaningful categories. But I find the system fairy complicated, and clinicians may be put off by its complex algorithms. The AMPD could run the danger of supporting the all-too-common practice of not diagnosing PDs at all. I suggest that the procedure for AMPD diagnoses in clinical settings needs to be simplified in order to make life easier for busy clinicians.

## BPD IN *ICD-11*

The *ICD-11* is the official classification system in medicine that is used around the world. Most diagnoses can be translated between *ICD* and *DSM* by using the same code. However, since the publication of *DSM-III* there have been some important differences between the *ICD* and the *DSMs*. The main one is that the *ICD* has never required the counting of criteria or used algorithms.

PDs show the most striking differences between the two systems. The experts who worked on *ICD-11* originally proposed that all categories of PD be removed and replaced with dimensional scores (measuring severity of psychopathology as well as trait profiles). Unlike the AMPD, though, these scores are not used to construct categorical diagnoses; instead, clinicians are asked to score five trait dimensions: negative affectivity, dissociality, anankastia (compulsivity), detachment, and disinhibition. Each of these dimensions can then be scored for intensity. The result is a profile. As I discuss later in this chapter, these dimensions closely resemble those in the AMPD and the FFM.

The plans for *ICD-11* led to major pushback from European and American researchers, some of whom have spent their professional lives studying BPD (Herpertz et al., 2017). Moreover, clinicians often find a diagnosis of BPD to be useful for treatment planning. In the end, a compromise was adopted. A "borderline pattern" was added to the trait profiles on the basis of descriptive paragraphs that are almost identical to the criteria for this category in *DSM-5*. In this way, a schism in the PD research community was avoided. But the architects of the *ICD-11* system continue to believe that BPD is a redundant construct, and they argue that a borderline pattern can account for the dimensions already described in that manual (Tyrer & Mulder, 2018). However, although several years have now passed since the adoption of *ICD-11*, the PD literature is still dominated by research papers on BPD as defined by *DSM*. The experts who devised the *ICD-11* system remain vocal in their opposition to that diagnosis, which they find too heterogeneous (Tyrer & Mulder, 2022).

Time will tell whether or not the *ICD-11* methods will be widely used in clinical practice. At this point, it is not happening. However, in spite of the contrary views of the experts who designed this system, the decision to maintain a borderline pattern in the manual was the right one.

## BPD AND TRAIT DIMENSIONS

The idea that PDs are best measured quantitatively as continuous dimensions has long been promoted by trait psychologists, who see PDs as pathological versions of normal traits (Krueger et al., 2018). They point out, correctly, that hypertension is a spectrum and that a blood pressure level of 140/90 is an arbitrary cutoff for diagnosis. On the other hand, clinicians still find it useful to view hypertension as a category, and they use a quantitative measure to assess its severity.

In the domain of personality psychology, the most influential and empirically supported schema is the FFM. This Big Five system uses questionnaire data to score patients on Extraversion, Neuroticism, Conscientiousness, Agreeableness, and Openness (Widiger & Costa, 2013). Thus, patients with BPD are high in Neuroticism (emotionally dysregulated) and low on Conscientiousness (impulsive). However, these traits do not fully account for problematic intimate relationships.

The FFM is based on the factor analysis of questionnaires that were given to large numbers of people in the community. Moreover, the five dimensions of the *ICD-11* model and the AMPD are very similar to the FFM factors. The main limitation of the FFM is that a method based on surveys administered to community populations may not be adequate for measuring pathological extremes seen in clinical practice.

Even so, some models go further and attempt to score all forms of psychopathology as dimensions. The HiToP system describes multiple levels of a hierarchy that range from an overall "p" (or psychopathology factor common to all disorders) to the symptoms that clinicians assess. This is an ambitious project, and several of the promoters of the AMPD were also listed as coauthors of the original HiToP article (Kotov et al., 2017). However, whereas the AMPD might be fully adopted on the basis of existing research, HiToP is still in the early stages of development, and it may not be ready for prime time.

The Research Domain Criteria framework (RDoC; Cuthbert & Insel, 2013) takes a different approach. Its dimensions are based on theory (mainly derived from neuroscience and cognitive sciences) rather than on factor analysis, and they range from neuronal networks to social stressors. RDoC has been strongly promoted by the National Institute for Mental Health, and it was intended to replace *DSM* categories in research. That has not happened. Also, RDoC is not, to my knowledge, currently being used in clinical settings. The main reason is that the neuroscience of mental disorders is in its infancy, cannot be measured in practice, and has thus far been unable to fully account for any form of psychopathology. Moreover, an emphasis on neuroscience downplays the crucial role of psychosocial factors in mental disorders (Paris & Kirmayer, 2016).

Another obstacle needs to be overcome before adopting dimensional systems. For psychiatry, it has always been important to remain a branch of medicine. The use of systems that are not recognizable by clinicians as diagnoses could widen the gap between psychiatry and other medical specialties. Clinical psychology could have less of a problem because it has traditionally focused less on targeting symptoms and instead has concentrated on disorders. Yet psychology research, over several decades, has also embraced the *DSM* system. Thus far, clinical psychologists who practice outside academic centers seem to prefer a categorical approach, as is used for diagnoses ranging from major depression to ADHD or PTSD. Clinicians will have to be trained to use the AMPD system. It may not be that hard do such training, but mental health professionals have thus far shown a lack of enthusiasm for making diagnoses on the basis of trait dimensions.

As of now, the *DSM* system, for all its problems, provides a common language for mental health clinicians. That is another reason why none of the alternatives to the *DSM* system have yet been widely adopted. For all of its problems, making a diagnosis of BPD remains important, because doing so leads patients to the best forms of treatment.

## COMORBIDITIES AND DIFFERENTIAL DIAGNOSIS

Because BPD is a mixture of pathologies derived from multiple domains, it has a high comorbidity with several other mental disorders. However, the very term "comorbidity" can be misleading if it is understood to mean that a patient has separate disorders. The way *DSM* is written, with similar symptoms in different categories, comorbidity is inevitable—but not always meaningful. Moreover, the system encourages clinicians, especially psychiatrists and family physicians, to treat multiple categories separately, which often leads to problematic treatment choices, such as polypharmacy. However, as I discuss in Chapter 4, it is an established fact that antidepressants have little effect on the core features of BPD. Thus, clinical psychologists are not missing anything if they are not in a position to prescribe medication for this disorder, and they may even be doing their patients a favor if they do not refer them to physicians (who are guaranteed to prescribe). It has also been reported that when BPD treatment is successful comorbid depression also goes into remission (Gunderson et al., 2004). The main exception to this overall conclusion is that severe substance abuse, eating disorders, or both may need separate treatment for these comorbidities.

### BPD, Depression, and Anxiety

Patients with BPD have a little bit of everything in the *DSM* manual. The list includes depression and anxiety, but these features are more chronic than episodic. As has long been observed, BPD patients suffer from depressed mood, but not in the same way as those who have a major depressive episode without a PD (Gunderson & Phillips, 1991). The difference is that mood in BPD is not time limited but is unstable and reactive to interpersonal conflicts. These rapid mood swings reflect a high sensitivity to the environment. In contrast, mood in depressive episodes, when severe, is relatively unresponsive to the environment. Moreover, mood swings in BPD are not episodes but often continue for years. These rapid changes are characterized by depression, anxiety, and/or rages. In fact, antidepressants are not very effective for mood symptoms in patients with PDs of any kind (Newton-Howes et al., 2006). You cannot medicate depression in BPD as if it were separate from the underlying personality pathology that drives it. How can one not be depressed if emotion dysregulation and impulsivity interfere with establishing a stable life? Unfortunately, psychiatrists and other physicians tend to prescribe antidepressants to almost all patients with BPD, wrongly believing that they can separate mood and treat it separately.

Moreover, mood swings in BPD are a clinical phenomenon that differs from major depression. These patients are highly sensitive to their environment, and if something positive happens mood can switch from low to high or even a bit high. Given the low bar for depression in the *DSM* (only 2 weeks of experiencing five out of nine symptoms), most patients with BPD will cross that threshold from time to time. And if you ask patients what they feel, they tend to describe chronic depression accompanied by anger; mood swings; and a sense of inner emptiness, hopelessness, and being cut off from the world. Research shows that when treatment targets BPD successfully, these depressive symptoms will remit (Gunderson et al., 2014).

The same limitation tends to apply to the use of cognitive behavior therapy (CBT) for BPD. Clinical psychologists trained in CBT could do better by integrating methods specific to BPD into their usual practice. Linehan (1993) developed dialectical behavior therapy because she found that CBT in its classical form was not sufficiently effective for these patients.

Self-harm, cutting in particular, is another signal that one is dealing with something more than episodes of depression. Not everyone who cuts meets criteria for BPD, but those who have the disorder are likely to do so (Reichl & Kaess, 2021). This behavior is often seen in adolescents, but it does not necessarily continue over the course of further development (Moran et al., 2012). Actually, self-harm that continues for months or years is a clue to the presence of emotion dysregulation (Biskin et al., 2021). Nonsuicidal self-injury can be confused with suicide attempts, yet cutting has a very different purpose. It relieves emotional pain, albeit temporarily, using behavior that is both distracting and physically painful (Nock, 2010).

Anxiety disorders are also common in BPD (Shah & Zanarini, 2018). Patients can have panic attacks or a chronic pattern of worry that characterizes generalized anxiety disorder. Those who are more introverted may also have a social anxiety disorder. However, as with depression, one cannot separate anxiety from personality, either in diagnosis or treatment. Standard methods of treating anxiety symptoms (medications and CBT) are generally less successful than interventions specific to BPD (Keuroghlian et al., 2015).

In summary, depression and anxiety are not separate from BPD and should not be treated as if they were. When BPD gets better, these comorbidities will remit.

CASE EXAMPLE 1.2
## DEPRESSION AND ANXIETY IN BPD

Claudia was a 19-year-old nursing student with a history of multiple visits to the ER for suicidal ideation. She had also been an intermittent cutter since age 15. Her severe mood swings were associated with rages during which she would scream and break things. Claudia also reported frequent panic attacks that did not remit with antidepressant medication. She had been a heavy cannabis user for several years, felt empty, and experienced dissociation and paranoid trends. Her relationships have been toxic and unstable. Claudia has had hookups when not in a relationship, as well as trouble being alone. When she has had a partner, that person tended to become the obsessive center of her life.

This case illustrates how depression and anxiety are part of a broader picture of mood swings, impulsivity, and unstable relationships.

### BPD and Bipolar Disorders

Because BPD patients have notable mood swings, some clinicians see these symptoms as a variant of bipolar disorder, falling within what has been termed a *bipolar spectrum* (Paris & Black, 2015). In addition, because some BPD patients also have brief psychotic episodes (lasting a few days at most), that makes the temptation to diagnose bipolarity even greater.

The most common form that is confused with BPD is not bipolar I disorder (with full mania) but bipolar II (with hypomania only). Because mood swings are common, the boundaries of bipolar II tend to be unclear. *Hypomania* describes a continuously elevated mood over at least 4 days, yet if you ask BPD patients about how long they feel high, the answer is almost always a few hours or, at most, a couple of days. Moreover, unlike bipolarity, where mood is not responsive to context, mood swings in BPD are driven by the environment. Moreover, the drugs used for classical bipolar illness are not effective for BPD (Paris, 2004). Finally, overlap with bipolar diagnoses may be an artifact of overly broad diagnostic criteria in small samples (Zimmerman & Morgan, 2013).

Unfortunately, it is not unusual to see typical cases of BPD for which psychiatrists or family physicians have been prescribing lithium or anticonvulsant drugs for years. This is a mistake given that mood swings do not necessarily fall within a bipolar spectrum. In BPD, they are part of the interpersonal sensitivity that characterizes the disorder. When these symptoms are treated as bipolar, patients do not benefit beyond an initial placebo response. Moreover, they can experience a side effect burden and may not be referred for evidence-based therapy.

There are a few patients in whom it is difficult to be sure whether they have bipolarity or BPD. This problem can arise when patients describe high periods that are reported to go on for longer than 4 days. But the length of mood episodes is not necessarily reported with accuracy by patients. Perhaps this overlap only reflects the way the *DSM* defines bipolarity and PDs.

Estimates of the frequency of bipolar symptoms in BPD patients have been rather variable, depending on samples, raters, and diagnostic biases. Reports of a 20% comorbidity with bipolar disorders (e.g., Gunderson et al., 2014) are dubious because they ultimately depend on reports from clinicians, many of whom favor a broad diagnosis of bipolar II. If a patient does not report a history of a continuous high that lasts for many days, and if the patient lacks characteristic features, such as a lack of any need for sleep, unwise spending, and changes in mood that have been observed by others, they probably do not have bipolar II disorder. If a conservative approach is taken, the differential diagnosis should not usually be difficult.

More recently, psychiatry seems to have regained its sanity, at least for now. Thus, misdiagnosis of BPD as bipolarity is less of a problem than it was 10 years ago. Perhaps this is because the message has gone out that BPD remits with time and is eminently treatable. One cannot say the same for bipolar disorders, which rank among the most difficult clinical problems in psychiatry and which can continue into old age.

CASE EXAMPLE 1.3

## DIFFERENTIAL DIAGNOSIS WITH BIPOLAR DISORDER

Doris was a 26-year-old woman working at a call center. She described mood swings during which she drove her car too fast and was sexually impulsive. These episodes usually went on for hours but could last as long as 2 to 3 days. During these periods, regular sleep was maintained even though she felt excited. In the past, Doris had been to the ER for suicidal ideation and had bouts of binge eating. She has been a cutter since early adolescence. Doris had been prescribed lamotrigine by her family physician, but with little benefit. She had been told by ER physicians that she had a bipolar disorder and considered that to be a definitive diagnosis. However, when informed by our clinic that she actually met criteria for BPD, she gained a new perspective on her problems.

This case is an example of how the presence of mood swings may lead to an incorrect diagnosis of bipolarity and how a broader view of symptoms from multiple domains can correct that error.

### BPD and Psychosis

Another pitfall in BPD diagnosis lies in the fact that some patients have brief psychotic episodes lasting a few days (Slotema et al., 2018), which may be seen as a form of mania or even schizophrenia. Patients with these symptoms need hospitalization and usually respond rapidly to antipsychotic drugs. However, unlike schizophrenia or bipolar I disorder, psychotic episodes in BPD are brief. (This may be the only scenario in which the term "borderline" is clinically meaningful.)

BPD patients more often have micropsychotic symptoms (Slotema et al., 2018). About half will hear critical voices, usually when under great stress from interpersonal conflicts. Visual hallucinations are more rare, often consisting only of seeing threatening black shadows. More often, patients with BPD have paranoid trends and can alternate between feelings of suspicion and naïveté. Much more common are dissociative phenomena involving depersonalization, or a feeling that the world is not real.

CASE EXAMPLE 1.4

## MICROPSYCHOTIC SYMPTOMS IN BPD

Ellen was a 25-year-old woman who worked for several years as a nurse. She was admitted to a psychiatry ward after presenting at an ER in a psychotic state, marked by the delusion that God had spoken to her and communicated to her a plan to save the world. During this time, which lasted for 72 hours, she heard voices instructing her about her mission. After receiving antipsychotic medication, Ellen recovered from this episode. She had no family history of bipolarity or psychosis. She did have a history of depression and self-harm going back to age 13, and she had presented several times to the ER with suicidal threats, usually after breakups with romantic partners. Her psychotic episode was therefore seen as a feature of BPD.

This case offers an example of the brief psychotic episodes seen in patients with BPD. These episodes can be distinguished from psychotic illness by their short duration and the presence of typical symptoms of a PD.

## BPD and ADHD

ADHD has recently become a popular diagnosis in adults, and the construct is broad enough that it can be seen as accounting for emotion dysregulation and impulsivity. There is a large body of research on ADHD in children (Barkley et al., 2010). One reason why it can be seen as having an overlap with BPD is the common factor of impulsivity. However, there are no biomarkers or psychological tests that can be used to definitively diagnose ADHD. Also, ADHD in adults usually fits the inattentive, rather than the hyperactive, subtype.

ADHD begins in early childhood, as is usually the case with neurodevelopmental disorders, and there is less controversy about its validity at that stage. But it is not sufficient to ask patients what they were like as children; validation may require reports from family members, report cards from teachers, and other sources. ADHD is now being diagnosed in adults who develop problems with focus or maintaining attention in adolescence, young adulthood, or later. It is well established that many cases of ADHD beginning in childhood can continue into adult life (Hechtman, 2016), but not all clinicians remember that if you follow the *DSM*, ADHD cannot be diagnosed in an adult without an onset prior to puberty. When problems begin later in development, other conditions, such as PDs, should be considered.

ADHD in adults may currently be the focus of what has been called a "diagnostic epidemic" (Frances, 2013; Paris et al., 2015). There has been concern about overdiagnoses that lead to overprescriptions (Kazda et al., 2021). In my own outpatient consultations, a very large percentage of patients ask me if they have this disorder, regardless of their symptoms, and some insist on receiving stimulants. These prescriptions have been becoming more frequent for some time (Olfson et al., 2013), and they are still increasing.

The problem is that there is no gold standard for an ADHD diagnosis. Even psychological testing, in spite of the heft of its reports and the cost of its procedures, is nonspecific and not always useful (Barkley, 2019). Ultimately, ADHD is a clinical diagnosis and, like many of the categories in the *DSM*, lacks a strong scientific basis in biomarkers. Moreover, attention problems in adults are ubiquitous and are associated with many other diagnoses.

Today, a large number of patients are coming to physicians with a self-diagnosis of ADHD that usually is based on what they have read on the web or have heard from friends. (The internet has been good for many things but bad in its tendency to promote self-diagnosis.) Many patients are looking for a prescription of stimulants, which they see as a cure for complex problems. Yet most people with ADHD symptoms that begin in adolescence or adulthood did not have it in childhood (Moffitt et al., 2015). It is possible that an adult onset reflects a different domain and a different diagnosis (Gascon et al., 2022). On the other hand, if there is a childhood onset pointing to a neurodevelopmental disorder, then treatment for ADHD in a minority of BPD patients might be considered. At this point, research does not give us an answer to that question. It would still not justify the vast increases in diagnosis of ADHD.

I have lived through many diagnostic fads over the course of my career, but the one for ADHD is one of the worst. If almost everybody has difficulties with focus, then a near-universal use of stimulants could become as uncontroversial as wearing eyeglasses. Something that is not widely known is that stimulants can increase focus in perfectly normal people, as first described almost 50 years ago (Rapoport et al., 1978). Thus, a positive response to medication does not prove that a patient has ADHD.

A lack of focus is associated with a wide range of mental disorders, most clearly with anxiety, depression, and PDs. Moreover, some people have more trouble focusing on tasks than others do, but they run into difficulty only when modern society requires them to sit in classrooms, or to have a desk job. The question is whether these problems are due to ADHD or to a mismatch between the ability to focus and the demands of modern society.

Finally, it is (or should be) common knowledge that placebo effects are strongly associated with the prescription of any drug, including stimulants (Benedetti, 2020). This could be why patients who take these agents tend to report a decrease in efficacy after a few months (Handelman & Sumiya, 2022). Moreover, there is little evidence that patients with BPD, regardless of whether they have problems with attention, can benefit from stimulants (research on this issue is rare). Once again, my best advice is to avoid the idea that comorbidity can guide therapy and to treat personality, not just symptoms.

---

CASE EXAMPLE 1.5

## DIFFERENTIAL DIAGNOSIS WITH ADHD

Estelle was a 30-year-old woman working as an administrative assistant. She reported a relatively normal childhood followed by serious adolescent turmoil (suicidality, self-harm, substance abuse, toxic relationships). These symptoms were less apparent in early adulthood, and although she only finished high school Estelle eventually came to work for an insurance company.

CASE EXAMPLE 1.5
**DIFFERENTIAL DIAGNOSIS WITH ADHD (*Continued*)**

When stressed by problematic attachments, she had great trouble focusing on her job. Estelle was not on medication of any kind, and she did not seek therapy. A friend suggested she might have ADHD, and her family physician referred her for a psychiatric assessment. Estelle referred to her problem as "my ADHD," which she saw as part of her identity. She was looking for a magic pill that would allow her to manage many complex problems. However, her later onset of symptoms was not consistent with that diagnosis, and her problems concentrating were more linked to the depression and anxiety that accompany BPD.

This case shows that problems with inattention and focus can have multiple origins in other disorders and on their own are not sufficient to diagnose ADHD.

## BPD and Autistic Spectrum Disorder

I find it puzzling that autistic spectrum disorder could ever be confused with BPD. Although patients in both of these groups can have emotion dysregulation, they are mostly the opposite of each other. A large-scale review (May et al., 2021) found no overlap between these diagnoses that exceeded the community prevalence of each of these categories. The only reason I can see for confusing autistic spectrum disorder with BPD is that it has recently been the subject of great diagnostic inflation (Paris, 2020a).

Admittedly, some BPD patients can be a bit peculiar and strange. But autism is a condition that begins in early childhood and interferes with the establishment of relationships across a lifetime. Patients on the autistic spectrum do not usually search for intimacy, and do not miss it when they do not have it, whereas BPD patients desperately seek close relationships.

As often happens when a spectrum is introduced, autistic spectrum disorder, like ADHD, is close enough to normality to be overdiagnosed (Frances, 2013). In fact, the diagnosis has become so popular that many patients wonder if they have it. It is sad, if somewhat understandable, that patients think they can diagnose themselves as well as trained clinicians can just by searching the internet. This is another example of how the web promotes simple (but often wrong) answers to complex questions.

## BPD, PTSD, and CPTSD

In this book, I present a critique of an all-too-common belief that BPD is mainly the result of psychological trauma during childhood. I will offer in its stead a biopsychosocial model in which childhood adversities interact with heritable traits, creating vicious cycles that lead to personality pathology.

A large-scale American community survey (Pagura et al., 2010) found that PTSD can be diagnosed in about 30% of patients who meet criteria for BPD—but this means that 70% do not have that diagnosis. Moreover, because the impact of trauma is such an emotional issue, even these numbers can be misleading, and it is important to distinguish between clearly traumatic events and growing up in a dysfunctional or unsupportive family. Following *DSM* criteria, a PTSD diagnosis requires specific symptoms (flashbacks and avoidance of triggers that bring back traumatic memories). Thus, although PTSD is a frequent comorbidity, the majority of BPD patients do not meet diagnostic criteria for PTSD. This is not surprising given that BPD is best understood in the context of a model in which trauma is important but is only one of many risk factors. It is also important to distinguish between trauma that occurs prior to the emergence of BPD (i.e., during childhood) from events that occur in adolescence or youth (e.g., sexual assaults or domestic violence) that may be, at least in part, consequences rather than causes of BPD.

The new diagnosis of CPTSD appears in *ICD-11*, but not in *DSM-5-TR* (which recognizes only severe PTSD). This construct is based on a theory that considers BPD a form of PTSD and that assumes that emotion dysregulation, impulsivity, and troubled relationships derive from multiple childhood traumatic events that interfere with adult development (Ford & Courtois, 2021).

The diagnosis of CPTSD has recently become very popular, even in countries like the United States and Canada, where the *DSM* system is usually preferred. One possible reason is that patients and their therapists prefer to embrace a model in which patients are seen as victims of unfortunate circumstances, as opposed to the view that they fall ill because they suffer more than others from exposure to adverse events. In this book, I argue that the CPTSD construct derives from assumptions that are not empirically supported.

Although a significant minority of patients with BPD have a history of childhood trauma, most people who have these histories do not develop BPD (Paris, 2020c, 2023c). A history of childhood trauma does not cause BPD, but it does make its course more chronic and severe (Soloff et al., 2008). Even so, many patients and therapists have embraced the CPTSD diagnosis. The most likely reason is that it moves the focus from problematic personality traits to experiences that are not seen as a patient's fault. I consider this defense of victimhood to be a false dichotomy because I adhere to an interactive model.

Once, when a colleague accused me of "not believing in trauma," my reply was that she did not seem to believe in genetic vulnerability.

---

**CASE EXAMPLE 1.6**

## DIFFERENTIAL DIAGNOSIS WITH PTSD

Flora was a 22-year-old woman presenting with suicidal ideation, self-harm, and intermittent substance use. She had left home at 18 because of a need to get away from a highly dysfunctional family. Her father was an alcoholic, and her mother was chronically depressed. She was often emotionally abused, occasionally beaten, and most certainly emotionally neglected. Flora supported herself by working in a veterinary clinic, where she had protective feelings for the animals, especially rescued ones. She was affected by her past and had great difficulty trusting other people. But Flora did not have symptoms such as flashbacks or being triggered to avoidance or distress by stimuli that could remind her of her childhood.

---

This case illustrates the context in which traumatic events are only one form of adversity that can increase the risk for BPD. These relationships are discussed in more detail in Chapter 3.

### BPD and Other PDs

Clinicians have become aware that BPD has a better prognosis than previously thought and that treatment is often successful. That is not the case for other forms of PDs. This may explain why some clinicians have followed a recent trend to overdiagnose BPD. They may see typical symptoms such as emotion dysregulation, suicide attempts, and/or self-harm, but many patients with these features may not meet formal criteria for BPD. Overdiagnosis occurs most often in patients who experience emotion dysregulation but lack the impulsivity and interpersonal problems that characterize BPD. These cases should be diagnosed as PD unspecified. For clinicians who use structured interviews, this is the most common diagnosis in practice, which emerges from a clinical picture that does not fit any PD category (Zimmerman et al., 2005).

BPD has been extensively researched, but most of the other *DSM* categories of PD have not (Paris, 2015). This is one of the main reasons why many trait psychologists prefer dimensional systems of diagnosis. And although it is likely that the methods of treatment developed for BPD are transdiagnostic, that hypothesis has not been fully tested. It therefore makes sense to offer such patients psychotherapy that was not designed for other PDs.

### BPD, Substance Use, and Eating Disorders

Substance use disorders are common and clinically important comorbidities in BPD (Trull et al., 2018). They are particularly common in men, which is one reason why we do not see as many male patients in the clinic as there actually are in the community (Trull et al., 2010). Lower levels of use of alcohol and cannabis use, below addictive thresholds, do not necessarily interfere with treatment in the way that heavy and consistent use does. Substance use is one of the few comorbidities that needs to be under control (usually through rehabilitation programs) before a patient starts therapy. The same can be said for problematic use of cocaine, amphetamines, and other drugs, such as opiates. Fortunately, most BPD patients are more likely to be simply users rather than actual addicts.

Similar considerations apply to eating disorders, which are more common in women than in men. Anorexia nervosa is associated with compulsive personality traits and is less common in BPD than impulsive patterns such as binge eating and bulimia nervosa (Steiger & Bruce, 2004). However, when bulimia (or mixed pictures of anorexia/bulimia) dominates the daily lives of patients, we may have to first refer these clients to an eating disorder program.

---

CASE EXAMPLE 1.7
## COMORBIDITY WITH SUBSTANCE USE

Grethe was a 27-year-old woman working in a clinic as a social worker. She had lost many jobs because of absences, most of which were related to binges on alcohol. Grethe has gone to rehab programs but always relapsed. She found Alcoholics Anonymous to be more depressing than helpful. She had also been seen in ERs for suicidal threats, and she has had many arguments with partners, usually when intoxicated. Grethe came to accept that she had a drinking problem, but she could never stop for more than a few weeks at a time. She was referred to a PD clinic but was told to get clean first and come back in 6 months when she was sober enough to be ready for therapy.

---

This case illustrates problems with a comorbidity that can derail treatment and therefore has to be managed separately and prior to therapy for

BPD. When patients are spending too much time on addictive behavior, this takes up the space for learning new skills.

## COMORBIDITY OR CO-OCCURRENCE?

Because PDs affect all aspects of psychological functioning, they are associated with a wide range of symptoms. As discussed in this chapter, however, PD, in particular BPD, is defined in part by a wide range of features that are better called *co-occurrences*.

High levels of co-occurrence of diagnosis are in part an artifact of categorical systems that inevitably lead to major overlap. A good thing to keep in mind is that the more co-occurrences you see in a patient, the more you should consider diagnosing BPD. Also, treatment methods that target particular symptoms can miss the point that psychotherapy treats a whole disorder and a whole person.

## SUMMARY POINTS

- BPD is a severe disorder that involves symptoms from multiple domains.
- The *DSM* system remains predominant, but there are other ways to diagnosis this disorder, including the AMPD, *ICD-11*, or the FFM.
- The comorbidities associated with BPD often lead to misdiagnosis, but some of them (especially substance use) tend to interfere with management.

# 2 PREVALENCE, PRECURSORS, AND OUTCOMES

Borderline personality disorder (BPD) is common in clinical settings as well as in the community. In this chapter, I examine research demonstrating that most cases of BPD begin in adolescence, and I explain the significance of that age of onset. I also review the long-term outcome of BPD, which usually involves partial or complete recovery in early adulthood. Although 5% to 10% of BPD patients eventually die by suicide (Paris, 2023b), the majority go on living and function at close to normal levels later in life.

## PREVALENCE OF BPD IN THE COMMUNITY

BPD is common both in the clinic and in the community. The best estimate of its clinical prevalence is that about 9% of personality disorder (PD) patients in a large outpatient setting meet *Diagnostic and Statistical Manual of Mental Disorders* (*DSM*; e.g., 5th ed., text rev. [*DSM-5-TR*]; American Psychiatric Association, 2022) criteria (e.g., for a BPD diagnosis; Zimmerman et al., 2005). The best evidence shows that its prevalence in community populations is close to 2% (Trull et al., 2010).

https://doi.org/10.1037/0000440-003
*A Concise Guide to Borderline Personality Disorder*, by J. Paris

These numbers probably fall in the right range, but they may not be precise. Epidemiological surveys in several countries, mainly in the United States, have estimated the prevalence of categories of mental disorders in the community by going door to door and interviewing representative samples (e.g., Kessler, Chiu, et al., 2005). In some ways, though, these procedures can be problematic. A large sample is required, but that means that research assistants, however well trained, have to collect the data, and researchers will use their reports for diagnostic evaluations. These problems could lead either to over- or underdiagnosis, in part because clinical features of *DSM* diagnoses tend to overlap and in part because diagnoses can be influenced by whichever categories are popular at any given time (Frances, 2013).

Moreover, survey methods do not easily establish a clear boundary between a disorder and normal problems in life. For example, major depression is so common that it has been called the "common cold of psychiatry." There is little doubt that depression is common worldwide (Vos et al., 2016). It is less clear whether its lifetime rate is as high as 15%, as some studies have claimed (e.g., Kessler et al., 1994). This would mean that one out of six people will suffer from clinical depression. The problem is that the bar for this diagnosis in the *DSM* system is low (5/9 criteria over a 2-week period). There is a difference between normal sadness and clinical depression, but it is hard to know where to draw the line. It might be better to label milder sadness not as a mental disorder but as unhappiness (Frances, 2013; Horwitz & Wakefield, 2007).

Surveying PDs in the community runs into a similar problem: What is the boundary between normal variations in trait profiles and diagnosable disorders? People with interpersonal problems may not think they have a PD, even when their family and friends have a different opinion. In fact, most surveys find that up to 12% of people in the community meet standard criteria for one of the *DSM*-defined PD diagnoses (Volkert et al., 2018). The rate for BPD is lower (close to 2%), but that is still a lot of people—several million in the United States alone.

A final issue is that because BPD came late to being recognized as a major public health problem, its prevalence only recently, in the past few decades, became the subject of research. This may explain why research findings of its prevalence have yielded divergent estimates. The highest prevalence, derived from a U.S. national survey of substance use, was 7% (Grant et al., 2004). That number is very doubtful because it differs from all the other surveys, and it is uncomfortably close to the clinical prevalence. All other studies have come up with much lower estimates: 1% in a British study (Coid et al., 2006), and 1.7% in the National Comorbidity Study (Lenzenweger et al., 2007). Unfortunately, there is a tendency to inflate the prevalence of mental disorders, mainly to encourage funding of research and treatment. For this reason, quite a few studies have quoted the misleading numbers in Grant et al.'s (2004) article. That estimate was later corrected by Trull et al. (2010) by setting a higher bar for diagnosis, reducing the community rate to 2%. Thus, a prevalence for BPD affecting somewhere in the range of 1% to 2% of the population is close to a consensus in research.

This level of prevalence is higher than the 1% rate for schizophrenia but similar to the 2% rate for bipolar disorders (Kessler, Chiu, et al., 2005; Kessler et al., 1994), but keep in mind that, like other mental disorders, BPD lies on a spectrum, and patients with it may or may not meet criteria at all times (Zanarini, 2019). At my clinic, we use a 2-year framework for diagnosis and add a structured interview (Zanarini et al., 1989) to narrow down the diagnosis and maximize its clinical relevance.

BPD may also vary from country to country or between cities and out-lying areas. One might think that this disorder is an urban phenomenon, but there is no evidence that BPD is any more common in large cities than in rural areas of the United States (Tomko et al., 2014). Although it would be useful to conduct parallel community surveys in developing countries, that has never been done, mainly because of a lack of funds. One can only say that cases can be identified in most clinical settings around the world (Paris & Lis, 2013). But BPD prevalence may be a moving target. As societies modernize around the world, their very structure could be a risk factor that could increase these numbers. This may be because modernity requires traits that favor individualism, whereas traditional societies are more collectivist and provide more social support (Kitayama et al., 2020).

Given that most BPD patients are female (Silberschmidt et al., 2015), one might assume that a similar gender ratio might apply to community populations, but most surveys have found that men and women have a similar prevalence, with only a small majority of females (Coid et al., 2006; Lenzenweger et al., 2007; Trull et al., 2010). The explanation for this discrepancy could be that women are more likely than men to seek help, in particular when experiencing mental disorders.

Finally, more cases of BPD are seen in lower than in higher socioeconomic populations (Ellison et al., 2018). That could be due to the fact that the disorder interferes with education or because of poverty, which lowers functioning in families, which is itself a risk factor. On the other hand, a survey conducted by Becker et al. (2023) found no differences by race but did show that sexual minority groups are more prone to the disorder.

## THE CLINICAL PREVALENCE OF BPD

The fact that the prevalence of BPD is much higher in clinical settings than in the community reflects the fact that patients seek treatment. But if many patients whom clinicians see in hospital clinics meet criteria for this diagnosis, how is it possible that BPD remained invisible for so long? (I never heard a word about this disorder in medical school.) There are several possible explanations. The first could be that its prevalence has gone up over time. There is indeed evidence that some of its symptoms (e.g., self-harm and substance use) have increased (Paris, 2020c). The second would be that patients with similar underlying pathology tend to develop different clinical symptoms at different times and places (Shorter, 1992). The third explanation would be that the increase is spurious and only reflects changes in diagnostic habits. A fourth possibility is that BPD has always been around but was not recognized. However, if that were the case, where are the case reports from the 19th or early 20th centuries that might support such a hypothesis? There are none.

In my opinion, the most likely explanation is the second one: that psychopathology, behind its current variations as diagnosable disorders, has a hidden inner structure that expresses itself with different symptoms at different time periods (Shorter, 1992). That point of view helps explain why certain diagnoses can spread by social contagion, both among clinicians and patients.

I also favor the view that BPD has been shaped in part by the demands (and problems) of modern society. We could test this idea by determining whether BPD has the same prevalence in different countries around the world, but all we have is a few case reports (Choudhary & Gupta, 2020). As noted, developing countries rarely have the resources to support epidemiological surveys. In Chapter 3, I discuss the conclusions about the clinical prevalence of BPD further.

In clinical settings, about 80% of BPD cases are females (Zlotnick et al., 2002). Males with BPD have a different pattern of comorbid disorders, marked by externalizing disorders, such as antisocial personality and substance abuse, whereas females with BPD have more comorbid internalizing disorders, such as depression and anxiety (Silberschmidt et al., 2015). (It has also been said that men do not like to ask for directions when lost, in the belief that doing so lowers their status.) Since the vast majority of the research and clinical work on BPD has focused on the majority who are female, this book will focus on women with the disorder.

Keep in mind that BPD, both in males and females, interferes with the capacity to commit to school and work when patients are young. Long-term follow-ups have shown that only about one-half of BPD patients ever have children (Paris & Zweig-Frank, 2001; Zanarini, 2019). However, those who do have children are probably less likely to die by suicide, given that the responsibility of being a parent is, for most people, a reason for living.

In spite of its tendency to remit over time, BPD is a major public health problem, taking up an inordinate amount of scarce human resources, mainly because of suicidality. As we will see, somewhere between 5% and 10% of these patients eventually die by suicide (Paris, 2023b). Yet access to treatment for BPD patients has always been difficult, and it remains difficult. This is unfortunate, given that therapy for this population is cost-effective (see Chapter 5).

One caveat: BPD, like other mental disorders, can have different levels of severity. Thus, the cases seen in clinics and outpatient practice are generally the most likely to remit as patients mature. However, the minority who do not remit can become major clinical problems. Because these cases tend to be the most visible, they can influence the way we see the prognosis of the disorder as a whole. The good news is that we have reasons to be optimistic about most of these patients, in whom BPD is largely a disorder of adolescence and young adulthood that usually remits in adulthood.

## PRECURSORS OF BPD AND ITS ADOLESCENT ONSET

BPD usually begins in adolescence, often in the years after puberty (Chanen et al., 2020; Chanen & McCutcheon, 2013; Videler et al., 2019; Winsper, 2021). This fact is not widely known because some clinicians are reluctant to commit to PD diagnoses that early, yet many major mental disorders begin at that stage of development. Because not all patients seek treatment, some cases do not reach a clinical level until mid- or late adolescence, sometimes coming to attention only months to years after initial symptoms appear (Zanarini, 2009).

Some of the most specific (albeit less severe) symptoms of BPD are common in adolescents. This is the stage when so many clinically significant features, such as mood swings, self-harm, and suicidal ideation, appear. Moreover, some cases begin even earlier in development. One longitudinal twin study found that BPD features can be identified as early as age 12 and are associated with other measures of severity (Wertz et al., 2020). A minority of patients may also describe suicidal ideas or attempts that occur before puberty (Janiri et al., 2020).

An onset of BPD around puberty is in accord with the fact that many teenagers have some degree of moodiness and impulsivity. However, only a few will self-harm or attempt suicide, and even among those who self-harm the course of such symptoms (usually cutting) tends to move toward remission (Moran et al., 2012).

An onset in adolescence contradicts the widely held (but incorrect) view that PDs cannot (or should not) be diagnosed before age 18. Actually, that rule (in *DSM-5-TR*) applies only to antisocial PD, and it was designed to separate cases in which conduct disorder remits (around age 18) from those in which antisocial behavior continues into adulthood. *DSM-5-TR* says that all other PDs can be diagnosed in adolescents if their criteria have been present for at least a year.

There is now a good deal of research on BPD in adolescence (Chanen et al., 2020). One survey found that its community prevalence at that stage of life is about 3% (Guilé et al., 2018), which is higher than the adult rate. This may be due to early remissions. My own group followed a group of patients who had been treated for BPD before age 18 (Biskin et al., 2011) and found that about one-half no longer met criteria by their early 20s. Early remissions in adolescence have also been documented by a longitudinal multisite study (Gunderson et al., 2003). These findings are consistent with a view of BPD as a disorder that begins after puberty but that has a variable age of remission.

Kaess et al. (2014) summarized these issues as follows:

> BPD has been a controversial diagnosis in adolescents, but this is no longer justified. Recent evidence demonstrates that BPD is as reliable and valid among adolescents as it is in adults and that adolescents with BPD can benefit from early intervention. (p. 782)

Moreover, some BPD symptoms in adolescence, in particular suicidal ideation and self-harm, may be on the increase (Reichl & Kaess, 2021).

Emotion dysregulation and impulsivity, marked by comorbidities such as substance use, bulimia nervosa, and promiscuous sexual behavior, may increase during the adolescent years (Chanen et al., 2020). The interpersonal aspects of adolescent BPD are also notable: One longitudinal study of girls found that those who were later diagnosed as having BPD already had premature and tumultuous romantic relationships (Lazarus et al., 2020).

One might ask whether there are childhood precursors of BPD that could allow for earlier interventions. Although the full clinical picture is rarely apparent in childhood, prepubertal symptoms, such as of conduct disorder and oppositional defiant disorder, can be precursors of BPD (Stepp et al., 2016). However, these are conditions that are not easy to treat. It is clear, though, that patients who develop BPD can experience significant levels of emotion dysregulation from an early age. These temperamental features, which lead to problematic emotions, can emerge in the form of mood swings later in development.

Many of the childhood and adolescent precursors to BPD were examined in a longitudinal follow up of nearly 2,500 prepubertal females, the Pittsburgh Girls Study (Stepp et al., 2014). One of its main findings was that the most significant predictors of adolescent BPD features (derived from parental and teacher reports) were high emotionality, high levels of activity, and low sociability, as well as shyness. However, because these are statistical findings it is not possible to predict outcome in individual cases. There is no single pathway leading to BPD.

Although many BPD patients describe growing up in a seriously dysfunctional family, the relationship of these risks to outcomes remains unclear (Yuan et al., 2023). Other patients report a normal childhood followed by explosive adolescent turmoil. This suggests that interactions between hormonal changes and psychosocial challenges can be a factor in triggering the disorder (Skabeikyte & Barkauskiene, 2021).

Keep in mind that dysfunctional families are a risk factor for a wide range of psychopathology and are far from specific to PDs (Paris, 2020a). Research in developmental psychopathology (Cicchetti & Rogosch, 2002) usually finds both *equifinality* (the same outcome from different risk factors) as well as *multifinality* (different outcomes from the same risk factors). These pathways indicate that there is no simple or linear relationship between risks and outcomes. Thus, if we cannot currently predict which children are at risk for BPD, we lack a useful guide for prevention. Moreover, documenting early adversities does not fully explain why young people develop this disorder. What clinicians may not always know is that children from dysfunctional families do not necessarily develop adult mental disorders (Fergusson et al., 2013; Rutter, 2012).

By the time adolescents are evaluated in clinical settings, they may have had serious problems for at least a year—something required by the *DSM-5-TR* for a diagnosis. However, these patients do not always seek help early on. Even when a diagnosis is clear, adolescents may be too impulsive to undergo therapy and attend sessions regularly (Choi-Kain & Sharp, 2012). A typical scenario involves multiple visits to the emergency room, after which patients may or may not follow through. Chanen (2015) recommended maintaining contact and watchful waiting until patients are ready to enter treatment programs. Fortunately, death by suicide under age 18 is much less common than at later ages (Cha et al., 2018). Although every adolescent suicide is always a tragedy, we need to keep its rarity in mind and focus on what suicidality tells us about emotion dysregulation.

The most important message of this research for clinicians is that BPD is fairly frequent among adolescents. Moreover, considering recent increases in self-harm at that age (Moran et al., 2012; Poudel et al., 2022), a clinical pattern of the full disorder may itself be on the increase. But if clinicians believe they cannot make a BPD diagnosis when patients are younger than 18, they may misdiagnose cases as depression or bipolarity, with the result that the patient will not be referred for specialized care specific to this disorder.

## BPD IN ADULTHOOD AND ITS LONG-TERM OUTCOME

The most common pattern for BPD in adulthood is for symptoms to peak in young adulthood, followed by a gradual recovery. Thus, most patients do not meet criteria after age 30–35 (Paris, 2003). In this respect, in spite of a clinically meaningful risk for death by suicide, BPD is a disorder with an overall good prognosis in the longer run. This view provides a better basis for optimism than many of the other diagnoses with which it has been confused.

Why, then, is BPD still seen by many mental health practitioners as chronic and intractable? This may be due in part to "the clinician's illusion": the tendency for patients who get better to stop coming while those who do not improve continue to seek treatment (Cohen & Cohen, 1984). This is the source of an misperception that patients are more chronic than they really are, a misperception that applies to BPD. The illusion of chronicity may be further strengthened by the clinical picture patients present in emergency settings, that is, when they are at their very worst. This having been said, not every patient fully remits, and a subgroup will experience chronicity (Zanarini, 2019).

These observations all support the view that BPD is most often a disorder that begins early in life and that gradually improves with time. An outcome of a partial or complete recovery has now been found in many studies, with both prospective and retrospective follow-ups. In the past, several retrospective cohorts were followed in research that examined outcomes after 15 years (McGlashan, 1986; Stone, 1990), and after 27 years (Paris & Zweig-Frank, 2001). All of these studies confirmed that most patients with BPD remit over time.

Similar trajectories of recovery have been documented in prospective research. The Collaborative Longitudinal Personality Disorders Study (CLPS; Gunderson et al., 2011) followed 175 BPD patients (as well as cohorts with other PDs and depression only) over 10 years. The McLean Study of Adult Development (MSAD; Zanarini, 2019) followed 290 BPD patients (compared with 72 who had other PDs) and collected data for 24 years. The findings of both studies showed that most patients improve with time and that many or most no longer met BPD criteria by their 30s, or even earlier. There were differences between these two samples; for example, patients in the

MSAD had been admitted to a psychiatric hospital, whereas CLPS patients, who were followed over 10 years, came from multiple sites at clinics based in university teaching hospitals. One reason why the 10-year follow-up of CLPS drew a more optimistic picture was that its sample was less severely ill at baseline, whereas the MSAD patients consisted entirely of those who had required hospitalization. This helps explain why the MSAD researchers found that even when patients no longer met criteria, many continued to experience psychosocial deficits 24 years later.

The discovery that BPD patients lose most of their symptoms over time was a surprise to many clinicians. Although the clinical features are most striking in youth, we do not see many of these patients once they approach middle age. In part, this pattern may be related to reductions in emotion dysregulation and impulsivity related to further brain development (which is not complete until around age 25). It is also possible that patients learn to avoid situations that make them dysregulated and impulsive. Some patients who do not currently meet criteria become socially isolated, in part because they know from past experience that intimate relationships trigger their symptoms.

The mood symptoms of BPD improve more slowly, but patients become less impulsive at an early point. (We are all less volatile in middle age than when we were young.) Findings concerning improvements in interpersonal relationships and the capacity to work in formal employment have been mixed. Most patients will achieve close-to-normal psychosocial functioning over time, but recovery is not necessarily complete, yet patients who drop out of school, and who do not work regularly, miss out on the developmental steps required to become a functioning adult. In relation to work, some doors will already have closed, and patients will need to make up for lost time.

Patients in middle age may continue to experience emotion dysregulation even if they no longer meet diagnostic criteria for BPD. Most of those who met the diagnostic criteria in their youth will mature and have reduced impulsivity, often avoiding life tasks (e.g., intimacy) as a way of staying out of trouble. The staff at our clinic use a 2-year time frame for diagnosis of a PD. If the criteria are not currently met, but serious problems remain, we may diagnose PD unspecified, or what can be called "lifetime BPD."

In a retrospective follow-up cohort (Paris & Zweig-Frank, 2001), about half of the patients had romantic partners at a mean age of 50, with a similar percentage having children. Their overall level of functioning in later middle age was quite variable, even though most were employed. Patients did better if they had a meaningful job or career, whereas chronic unemployment was associated with a poorer outcome.

Follow-up studies have demonstrated recovery for most patients with BPD, but a minority continue to struggle with close relationships and work. Overall, the reputation of BPD for being intractable turns out to be wrong. Even if that was a surprise, it was a pleasant one. After a gradual recovery, most patients no longer met criteria after age 30 to 35. In this respect, in spite of a clinically meaningful risk for suicide, BPD has a good prognosis in most cases, and this diagnosis provides a better basis for optimism than many of the disorders with which it has been confused.

The clinician's illusion, that patients appear to be more chronically ill than they really are, is evident here. This perception may be further strengthened by how patients present in emergency settings, that is, when they are at their very worst. This does not square with evidence showing that BPD usually, albeit gradually, improves with time. Some experts (e.g., Livesley, 2017) have attempted to predict outcome by defining subgroups of patients on the basis of severity of dysfunction. However, research has not found strong predictors (Herzog et al., 2020). The outcome of BPD is heterogeneous: Some patients do surprisingly well, whereas others retain a disappointing level of chronicity.

How can we explain why the clinical features of BPD are so striking in youth but so much less common in middle age? These changes may be partly related to reductions in impulsivity related to further brain development—which, keep in mind, are not complete until around age 25 (Mitchell, 2020). Patients can also learn from experience. Both of these changes promote better emotion regulation. Many patients will also, over time, avoid situations that make them dysregulated and impulsive. However, keep in mind that some who no longer meet BPD criteria can become socially isolated because they know that intimate relationships can trigger symptoms.

Findings about long-term outcomes for managing intimacy and the capacity to work have been mixed. Most patients will achieve close to normal psychosocial functioning over time, but recovery is not necessarily complete. Keep in mind that patients who drop out of school, and who do not work regularly, have missed the steps during adolescence that are needed to become a functioning adult. Some doors will already have closed, and patients need to work hard to make up for lost time.

In one cohort (Paris & Zweig-Frank, 2001), the majority of participants (59 out of 64) no longer had BPD in middle age. Although only half were living with a partner, in this population being single is not necessarily a detriment. Patients who had friends, a community of some kind, as well as a meaningful career, had a better outcome. Although BPD patients in middle age are less impulsive, a few still look for treatment if they continue to be emotionally dysregulated. This picture of partial recovery might be described as "graduating" from BPD to PD unspecified. On the other hand, some of these patients become isolated to the point of becoming locked into a more avoidant pattern.

Keep in mind that retrospective and prospective research designs do not necessarily yield representative samples. Retrospective follow-ups do not find everyone, and only some respondents will sign up for a prospective follow-up. Moreover, BPD is a heterogeneous disorder in which initial severity may or may not predict long-term impairment. More research is needed to find better predictors of outcome in this disorder.

Finally, it is important to note that not all BPD patients are the same. As Livesley (2017) noted, some remain in the community, do not seek treatment, and are functioning relatively well. Others seek outpatient treatment but have never been hospitalized, whereas those who have been hospitalized will not have been functioning well at baseline and have a more guarded prognosis. Fortunately, the majority of patients clinicians see will require only outpatient therapy.

In summary, most follow-up studies demonstrate that recovery is the most frequent outcome for patients with BPD but that a significant minority continue to struggle with managing close relationships and work. In spite of these variations in outcome, though, the reputation of BPD for being intractable is clearly wrong.

---

CASE EXAMPLE 2.1

## FULL RECOVERY FROM BPD

Helen was a 20-year-old student who presented to the emergency room with suicidal threats. She had taken several overdoses in the past and had a long-standing pattern of self-harm. Helen was raised by an alcoholic single mother and had little family support. She was seen in psychotherapy for 6 months, after which she improved sufficiently to be discharged.

Helen was reevaluated 15 years later as part of a follow-up study. By that time, she no longer had any of the symptoms of BPD. She was married, with two children, and had a stable job as a social worker. Helen looked back on her adolescence as a period of turmoil that was now well behind her. With many things to live for, she was no longer considering suicide.

---

This case is typical of a full recovery from BPD. In such cases, one may only see a mild level of emotional instability or dysregulation.

The next case examples describe a minority of patients who do not respond well to treatment and who go on to withdraw from life as a way of coping with emotion dysregulation triggered by interpersonal conflict. These patients will still have a PD, but they lack meaningful relationships.

CASE EXAMPLE 2.2
## PARTIAL RECOVERY FROM BPD

Irene was a 35-year-old woman working as a nurse, a job she enjoyed. She was divorced and lived with her 10-year-old daughter. Although Irene had been suicidal in the past, in view of her responsibility as a mother she considered that option to be off the table. She had stable friendships and felt there was no reason why she needed a man in her life. On the few occasions when she had dated, she felt her emotions go out of control and would not proceed further.

This case is typical of a partial (but meaningful) recovery, in which emotion dysregulation came under control, making it possible to see improvements in other domains of functioning.

CASE EXAMPLE 2.3
## FAILURE OF RECOVERY FROM BPD

Jasmine was a 45-year-old woman with multiple admissions for suicidality and BPD during adolescence and young adulthood. Jasmine had mostly toxic relationships in the past, and currently did not have a partner, or any children. She had been in multiple therapies, and had been tried on many antidepressants, but did not feel that talk therapy or medication helped her very much. For this reason, she no longer actively sought treatment. She spent her days at home, living mostly online, and when she went out she talked only to a few people she knew, at her local mall. Although Jasmine was still unhappy, she had only passive suicidal ideation.

This case is typical of a failure to recover, accompanied by a move into the territory of an unspecified PD.

## OUTCOME OF SUICIDALITY IN BPD

Let us now examine how often BPD patients, after years of chronic suicidality and suicide attempts, end up dying by suicide. The answer is that in spite of being suicidal for years on end, most will not die by suicide.

Suicide rates in BPD differ in different samples. Several retrospective studies (Paris & Zweig-Frank, 2001; Stone, 1990) have reported rates close to 10%, although others have noted a lower rate (McGlashan, 1986). One meta-analysis estimated an overall suicide rate of about 8% (Pompili et al., 2005). Although a meta-analysis of several prospective studies found a lower rate, it is best to rely on the largest research programs. In the CLPS study, the rate was 6% (Gunderson et al., 2011), about the same as in the MSAD cohort (Temes & Zanarini, 2018).

The main limitation of using prospective cohorts is that samples differ in severity at baseline. Thus, patients who sign up for research studies may be less likely to die by suicide. It is therefore difficult to say which of these numbers is representative of the larger patient population. What is clear is that at least 90% of BPD patients, in spite of years of chronic suicidality, never die by their own hand (Paris, 2023b).

It is also notable that most suicides occur later in the course of BPD and are less common among the younger patients seen in emergency rooms. In one of my own samples, the mean age at suicide was 38 (Paris & Zweig-Frank, 2001). That was the most important finding. It confirms that suicide does not usually occur in youth (when threats are most common) but later in development, usually after many failed treatments. In fact, suicide in BPD is more likely to occur after treatment than during psychotherapy. One explanation could be that suicide is more likely after a series of unsuccessful interventions, leading to a feeling of hopelessness, yet there is no way of making useful clinical predictions as to which patients will eventually die by suicide. The vast majority of patients, however ambivalent, still want to live, and they use suicidality as a way of communicating distress (Paris, 2023b).

There is another way that BPD affects longevity. Up to 14% of BPD patients have a shorter life span, losing up to 10 years compared with people who do not have this disorder (Fok et al., 2014), and they are more likely to die from medical causes than from suicide (Temes et al., 2019). My colleagues and I reported very similar findings in a retrospective cohort (Paris & Zweig-Frank, 2001). The most likely reason for this is that many patients continue to be impulsive, use substances, gain weight, and do not seek adequate medical care.

Research on the course and outcome of BPD has shown that patients with BPD usually recover and that relatively few will die by their own hand.

These findings have encouraged therapists to take on these challenging patients. The majority will benefit from treatment, and even those who do not will usually improve with time. However, some patients remain chronically suicidal for a longer time. I return to this issue in Chapter 6, where I discuss possible approaches to this difficult clinical problem.

## SUMMARY POINTS

- BPD affects about 2% of the people in community populations, but it is much more common, because of treatment seeking, in clinical populations.
- BPD usually emerges in adolescence and can be diagnosed at that stage.
- BPD gradually remits in most cases prior to middle age; however, some patients remain chronic and low functioning.

# 3 A BIOPSYCHOSOCIAL THEORY OF BORDERLINE PERSONALITY DISORDER

Borderline personality disorder (BPD), like most mental disorders, can best be understood in the context of a biopsychosocial (BPS) model. In this model, a biologically based vulnerability interacts with negative life experiences. For BPD, the best supported hypothesis is that heritable emotion dysregulation is made worse by emotional neglect, leading to clinical symptoms. In this chapter, I also explain why a posttraumatic theory of BPD is not correct, although severe childhood trauma does worsen the prognosis of the disorder.

## THE BPS MODEL

Nearly 50 years ago, the psychiatrist George Engel (1977) introduced the BPS model to conceptualize the causes of illness in medicine, and he went on to show that this theory can be applied to mental disorders (Engel, 1980). BPS theory hypothesizes that almost all forms of psychopathology have multiple causes that interact with each other. The model states that neither biological factors (e.g., genes or brain circuitry), nor psychological factors (e.g., trauma or other life adversities), nor social factors (e.g., stressors related

https://doi.org/10.1037/0000440-004
*A Concise Guide to Borderline Personality Disorder*, by J. Paris

to living in a particular culture or society) can, by themselves, explain why people develop mental disorders.

All mental disorders have a biological component that, in interaction with environmental factors, underlies a vulnerability to psychopathology. Yet although these factors have been studied using the methods of genetics and neuroscience, biology is not the only cause of mental disorders but instead comprises risk factors for their development. Thus, genetic and neural variations have statistical correlations with psychopathology, but they do not necessarily predict it. Although some traits or biological markers are associated with an increased risk for many disorders, most people with these profiles will never become ill. Given a reasonable environment, these variations can often be adaptive. That is why these traits have not been eliminated by natural selection.

The role of heritable traits is reflected in *temperament,* a term that describes behavioral and emotional characteristics present at birth that determine how people react to their environment (Rutter, 2006). The effects of these risks can be understood only by considering interactions between life adversities and genetically driven temperamental variations. That explains why problematic traits remain in the gene pool. By themselves, risk factors do not necessarily lead to mental disorders, but they do lead to a range of variations in emotion, behavior, and cognition.

These principles have been supported by research in behavioral genetics (Fuller & Simmel, 2023; Jang, 2005). With a behavioral genetics method, one can compare identical and fraternal twins to measure concordance, either for specific symptoms or for full diagnoses. Differences between monozygotic and dizygotic twins is the basis for a quantitative estimate of heritability that can be calculated from this information. These numbers can be converted into percentages that describe the overall likelihood of an outcome in a community population.

The most severe forms of psychopathology, such as psychoses, can have heritability as high as 80%, whereas the more common disorders, such as depression and anxiety, tend to have a heritability of about 40% (Jang, 2005). Most mental disorders will not develop without an additional environmental component. But to the surprise of many, the environmental factors in mental illness are *unshared* (not related to growing up in the same family) rather than *shared* (related to growing up in the same family). This means that children in the same family need not necessarily develop the same form of psychopathology and that siblings who grow up together may have no mental disorder at all. Instead, the most important environmental risks are life events that are unique to an individual and not to a family.

In the same way, life adversities by themselves do not explain the origins of personality disorders (PDs). Like depression and anxiety, the heritability of BPD is about 40% (Jang, 2005). This means that some people are more vulnerable than others because of underlying temperamental characteristics and that different people react differently to the same environmental challenges.

However, estimates of heritability cannot be applied to individuals. They are averages derived from populations, so some patients may have a higher level of heritability while other others have a lower level. Moreover, there is another biological pathway to psychopathology, which consists of random effects derived from how neurons make connections during embryonic development and childhood (Mitchell, 2020).

As a result of these effects, BPD patients tend to have a problematic temperament that makes them more vulnerable to adverse life events. These individual differences have sometimes been referred to as a contrast between orchids and dandelions (Boyce, 2019). A similar idea has been called *differential susceptibility to the environment* (Belsky & Pluess, 2009). But there is a twist in the story that helps explain why heritable traits of this kind remain in the population: People who are susceptible to negative events are also unusually responsive to positive events.

I am often asked to explain these principles to patients who ask me what causes BPD. I tell them they may have had a hard time in life but that they have always been more sensitive to stressors, more prone to get upset, and to have trouble calming down. The good news is that people can learn how to control dysregulated emotions.

In summary, although there are environmental risk factors in almost all mental disorders, they do not by themselves lead to psychopathology; instead, adversities most strongly affect those who are vulnerable and have less influence on those who are not. For this reason, there is no such thing as a mental disorder entirely caused by life events—not even posttraumatic stress disorder (PTSD), which also has a heritable component (McNally et al., 2015); instead, patients are most likely to develop symptoms when exposed to interacting biological, psychological, and social risk factors.

## GENETICS, TRAUMATIC EVENTS, AND SOCIAL STRESSORS

I have written a book about how BPS theory can be applied to psychological trauma, and in this section I briefly summarize its conclusions (Paris, 2023a, 2023c). It is a myth that trauma, by itself, is a consistent cause of mental disorders. Even in PTSD, adverse events lead to symptoms in only about 5% to 10% of those exposed. Thus, PTSD is not an inevitable outcome of exposure to adversity but reflects interactions between temperamental sensitivity and stressful events. A BPS model is needed to account for disorders associated with heritable traits, life adversities, and an unsupportive environment. This principle applies to all mental disorders. Thus, traumatic events do not account for the specificity of any mental disorder, which is largely determined by predispositions. What follows is that to understand trauma, you need to know something about genetics.

Trauma is, of course, a risk factor for certain outcomes, but it is only one of many risks that interact with each other (McNally et al., 2015). It is true that in complex systems, a single factor can trigger a cascade (Wichers et al., 2019), but that is not the same thing as making a potential trigger into a single cause.

Moreover, a history of traumatic exposure is highly nonspecific. It raises the risk for almost every mental disorder, including psychoses (Barrigón et al., 2015). Trauma is also a risk factor for physical illnesses of all kinds, such as heart disease (Krantz et al., 2022).

The risk for PTSD is strongly related to high levels of the personality trait of neuroticism (Paris, 2023a). Like all traits, neuroticism has a moderately large heritable component of about 40% (Widiger & Costa, 2013). Put simply, some people are more strongly affected by stressors than others. Neurotic traits remain in the gene pool because they are protective in the face of real danger. But higher reactivity can also lead to gene–environment interactions that start vicious cycles. That is the case for patients who develop BPD, who have high levels of trait neuroticism (Paris, 2020c). As I discussed in Chapter 1, however, although PTSD can be found in many cases of BPD, it is not present in the majority of cases.

We also need to consider the effects of social factors in the etiology of mental disorders; however, these relationships are not simple. The idea that social stressors such as poverty or racism, by themselves, can cause illness confuses risk factors with causes. A poor social environment also raises the risk for many negative outcomes but is not, by itself, a primary cause of mental disorders (Brüne, 2001). It has been suggested that BPD can also be understood in an evolutionary context. Thus, a fast lifestyle, which we see in patients who are highly emotional and impulsive, is an adaptation to an unpredictable social environment (Brüne, 2016)

Although the most severe forms of psychopathology are fairly universal, some mental disorders have symptoms that are variable over time and cultures (Bhugra et al., 2022). For example, classical hysteria (with conversion symptoms) was common in the 19th century, but we rarely see this clinical picture today. Instead, patients are presenting more often with PDs. Moreover, symptoms that are socially sensitive, such as eating disorders and self-harm, have become more frequent as traditional societies modernize and adopt Western values (Paris, 2020b). To consider a recent example, technological changes, in particular a widespread use of the internet, may be affecting adolescents in a way that leads to a range of problematic feelings and behaviors (Twenge, 2023). Once again, though, such risks have a stronger effect on those who are biologically and psychologically vulnerable.

Notably, some of the symptoms that have been on the increase in the general population in recent years include self-harm and suicidality, which can be hallmarks of BPD. A process of social contagion within social networks may be affecting the prevalence of these features (Jarvi et al., 2013). It is possible that as our culture becomes more problematic and less supportive of certain trait profiles, BPD could be on a trajectory to having a higher prevalence.

## APPLYING THE BPS MODEL TO BPD

BPD has a complex etiology. The key feature of the disorder is emotion dysregulation, such that this can be seen as an amplification of a vulnerable and environmentally sensitive temperament (Choi-Kain et al., 2017). BPD patients have intense and unstable reactions to psychosocial stressors, leading to intense emotions associated with mood swings and/or rages. Emotion dysregulation also promotes impulsive behaviors and troubled relationships. All these components of BPD, when studied separately, have been shown by behavior genetics research to be moderately heritable (Chapman, 2019). Then, gene–environment interactions produce what cancer researchers have called a *double hit*. That process leads to a feedback loop, with intense reactions to life stressors leading to more dysregulated behaviors, which then promote even more dysregulation.

Most clinicians accept that interactive mechanisms help account for mood disorders, anxiety disorders, and psychoses, yet BPD is not always understood in the same way. If the disorder is seen as mainly biological, patients with mood swings may be misdiagnosed as falling within a bipolar spectrum. If seen as mainly psychosocial, BPD can be misdiagnosed as a form of PTSD (or complex PTSD; see Chapter 1). Instead, we need to think about BPD in terms of gene–environment interactions. Impressed by the drama of a traumatic history, clinicians may be attracted by the simplicity of seeing BPD as almost entirely the result of an adverse childhood. This oversimplification has encouraged a belief that childhood trauma, by itself, is the main cause of the disorder.

Some recent research has supported the conclusion that the relationship between childhood trauma and BPD is at least in part genetically mediated. One study (Skaug et al., 2022) followed twins who were discordant for BPD and concluded that exposure to trauma in childhood and/or adolescence did not necessarily lead to a later development of the disorder and that the association between trauma and BPD can be best accounted by genetic influences. In this light, the risk for BPD and reacting strongly to life events may be much the same.

These findings are consistent with research that my colleagues and I have conducted on siblings (Laporte et al., 2011). We compared 56 BPD female patients with their sisters and found that in spite of growing up in the same family, only three sibling pairs were concordant for BPD. We concluded that one cannot explain the development of the disorder without considering gene–environment interactions. Keep in mind that, as a recent review of trauma and BPD emphasized (Yuan et al., 2023), all findings concerning the role of trauma in psychopathology are correlations that cannot prove causality. Longitudinal studies of twins (Bornovalova et al., 2009, 2013; Wertz et al., 2020) have come to the same conclusion.

Porter et al. (2020) conducted a meta-analysis of all studies of childhood adversity as risk factors for BPD and found that the most specific relationships with that outcome were not with traumatic events but with emotional neglect (what in dialectical behavior therapy is called *failure of validation*) and emotional abuse (constant criticism). There is much less research on emotional abuse, but it seems likely that families that are neglectful of emotions will be overly critical.

The main reason why the traumatic theory of BPD is misleading is that it does not explain why most people with trauma histories do not develop the disorder. This is not to say that trauma plays no role but that it needs to be more narrowly defined to separate neglect from abuse. Keep in mind that genes also have a strong effect on parenting behaviors, with traits shared at a 50% level between parents and children (Oliver et al., 2014). This theory also entirely fails to consider genetic factors in development.

Finally, traumatic theories may not be helpful for patients if they are encouraged to see themselves as victims of adversity (Paris, 2023b). Introducing genetics into etiological formulations in no way leads to blaming the victim. One can validate past experiences without blaming everything that goes wrong in a person's adult life on adverse life events.

Therapists also should not ignore genetics because doing so is seen as leading to hopelessness. This view is not correct. Consider that some of us have perfect vision, but many of us need to wear glasses. Similarly, we are all different in temperament, but some of us are extroverts, and some are introverts, and people vary greatly in levels of neuroticism. We adapt our lifestyles to these variations in personality. That is one of the tasks of psychotherapy for PDs.

In summary, even the most severe trauma does not always have a seriously negative impact. Its effect on later functioning is statistical but not consistent. Most people are resilient to adversity, and trauma may also lead what is called *steeling* (Rutter, 2012). For example, an ability to understand emotions in ourselves and others may emerge from a troubled childhood. One recent review (Bryce et al., 2023) found that people who have had adverse early life experiences are more likely to choose helping professions (e.g., psychotherapy).

## BIOLOGICAL FACTORS IN BPD

Let us now take a more detailed look at what research tells us about the biological factors in BPD. It is similar to most mental disorders in that heritable factors account for about 40% of the variance (Amad et al., 2014). Because heritability is averaged across a population, this does not mean that every patient carries the same genetic risk. What it does mean is that, as with other mental disorders, affected patients carry a temperamental risk for this form of psychopathology.

The precise nature of the genetic risk in BPD patients remains obscure. The evidence certainly suggests that it has something to do with failure of the prefrontal cortex to control activity in the limbic system (Niedtfeld & Bohus, 2019). But there is no such thing as a gene or a set of genes for BPD. We can document this complexity by examining the results of genome-wide association studies, which add up influences from the entire genome (Tam et al., 2019). This kind of research requires large samples but can document what has been called a *heritability gap* in that, although up to half of most disorders is influenced by heritable factors, genetic correlations explain only 5% of the variance (Fuller & Simmel, 2023). The same conclusion applies to BPD (Witt et al., 2017). This means that our current methods are insufficient to understand the complex interactions of genes.

Genetic effects on development do not arise from changes at one allele, or at just a few sites, but from interactions between very large numbers of sites.

And because genes have only a statistical relationship to outcome, genomic research can never fully explain the causes of non-Mendelian, highly polygenic forms of psychopathology. For this reason, decoding the genome has not attained the value for medicine that was expected of it just a few decades ago. The idea that mapping genomes to personalize treatment of mental disorders (as is being tested for some forms of cancer) remains unrealistic for now.

It is also true that genes influence behavior through synaptic pathways governed by chemical transmissions that carry signals to the synapses, but there no such thing as a chemical imbalance that explains psychopathology in mental disorders (Moncrieff et al., 2023), or specifically for BPD. The once-popular theory that serotonin, or another neurotransmitter, is the key to disorders characterized by moodiness and impulsivity is far too simplistic.

Researchers have long hoped to use the technology of brain scans to assess neurophysiology. Some of these studies have shown changes in volume and/or in activity in specific regions (Herpertz & Bertsch, 2022). Such findings support the hypothesis that a lack of control of emotions and behaviors is associated with a failure of inhibition of limbic system activity (Krause-Utz et al., 2017). However, these associations remain too nonspecific to serve as a reliable biological marker for BPD.

To put this issue into perspective, we are far from finding biomarkers for any major mental disorder. The same is true for the biology of BPD, for which the data are at best suggestive. Moreover, the genetic factors behind temperamental vulnerability in these patients are almost certain to be highly complex. Those who have claimed, again and again, that we are on the cusp of a breakthrough have not met our expectations. They underestimate the complexity of the human brain, with its 86 billion neurons and 100 trillion synaptic connections.

A systematic review of Linehan's (1993) biosocial model (Crowell et al., 2009) concluded that although the theory was conceptually strong, it needed much more investigation. Niedtfeld and Bohus (2019) summarized a large body of neurobiological evidence consistent with the conclusion that BPD patients have variations in brain connectivity that make them more prone to emotion dysregulation. These problems are also associated with deficient emotion recognition (Domes et al., 2009) as well as emotional avoidance (Schramm et al., 2013). Research points to a relationship between emotion dysregulation and deficits in specific neuroanatomical pathways, such as the anterior cingulate cortex, amygdala, and insula (Ruocco et al., 2010), as well as limbic overactivity (Koenigsberg, 2010). Overall, this line of investigation suggests that a failure of the frontal lobe to modulate limbic input leads to emotion dysregulation. These variations in brain activity are almost certainly under genetic influence. Consistent with this assumption, behavioral genetics research has shown that all traits are at least partially heritable (Turkheimer, 2000).

Decades ago, data from a large community sample of twins, using a self-report measure of affective instability, found that unstable mood has the same moderate levels of heritability as BPD itself (Jang et al., 1996). More recently, Hawn et al. (2015) reviewed twin studies that also showed a moderate estimate of heritability for emotion dysregulation, similar to what is found in internalizing disorders. However, BPD presents with a mixture of externalizing and internalizing features. These conclusions are further supported by research showing that BPD has a heritable component that accounts for 45% to 50% of the variance (Amad et al., 2014). Beauchaine and Cicchetti (2019), in their summary of behavior genetics studies, also observed that all BPD-associated trait dimensions are linked.

The molecular mechanisms behind trait vulnerability are unknown. Although behavior genetics methods yield overall estimates of heritability, they do not tell us how phenotypic differences are linked to genes. Once the genome was decoded, a research program set out to identify specific genes for specific traits or forms of psychopathology, but the search for candidate genes was not in any way successful. Now, with the development of genome-wide association studies, we can examine the genome as a whole (Assary et al., 2018). However, this method shows that most phenotypes of mental disorder are influenced by hundreds or thousands of alleles (Tam et al., 2019). This is a level of complexity that could be handled only by artificial intelligence.

## PSYCHOLOGICAL FACTORS IN BPD

A large body of research on BPD patients supports the view that early adversity is common in this population (Paris, 2020c). However, meta-analyses have shown that the most important risk factors in family life for the later development of BPD are emotional neglect and emotional abuse (Porter et al., 2020). However, the view that childhood trauma is the main cause of the disorder (as well as of many other forms of psychopathology) remains popular. Promoted by best-selling books (e.g., van der Kolk, 2015) and by the drama required for cinema, this idea has gripped the imagination of patients, clinicians, and the general public. These ideas have even been used to create a domain of psychology called *traumatology*. But the idea that adverse experiences always make people sick is not supported by research.

Research also has failed to show that trauma is not the main cause of any mental disorder. That includes PTSD, in which symptoms develop in only 5% to 10% of those exposed to severe life adversity (Paris, 2023c). The story is similar in BPD. Childhood trauma is common, but although traumatic events contribute to severity they are far from universal in the life histories of patients (Porter et al., 2020). Moreover, only a minority of traumatized children go on to develop the disorder (Paris, 2022b). Thus, although childhood trauma certainly plays a role in the risk for BPD, it is not its main or only cause.

We have been misled by overly inclusive definitions of "trauma," which are sometimes used to describe almost any kind of early adversity. Moreover, correlation does not add up to causation. An emphasis on trauma has also led to a kind of redefinition of BPD as a form of complex PTSD (Paris, 2023a), yet the use of the word "complex" may actually avoid acknowledging complexity given that it does not account for the heritable factors in this disorder.

Trauma is a risk factor for a wide range of psychopathology, but it is not specific to any single diagnosis. Moreover, as already noted, traumatic theories do not explain why, as shown by longitudinal follow-up studies of children, the majority of those who experience serious adversities early in development do not develop mental disorders, including PDs (Bulbena-Cabre et al., 2018). I have summarized this literature in two books that examine the roles of genes and environment in mental disorders and, more generally, in personality development (Paris, 2020a, 2022a). Here I would like to pay homage to the late British psychiatrist Michael Rutter (2006), who pioneered an interactive and multivariate approach to the understanding of psychopathology in children and adolescents.

Rutter (2012) was also a pioneer in the study of resilience. On the basis of a large body of research that used longitudinal designs to study human development, the conclusion with the strongest evidence base is that resilience is the rule, not the exception. Clinicians can misjudge the role of psychological risk factors if most of the people they see have symptoms and behaviors. They do not see the large number of people who have endured similar experiences and have not developed mental disorders. That is why research in the community is important for putting clinical impressions into context.

The idea that trauma is the main cause of BPD also derives from a misinterpretation of life histories. A notable minority of patients have experienced serious neglect and family dysfunction, sometimes to the point of requiring child protection services. Again, what research has actually shown is that a traumatic history leads to higher levels of symptoms and interferes with recovery (Soloff et al., 2002). Thus although childhood trauma is statistically associated with poor outcomes (Norman et al., 2012), it covaries with emotional neglect. There is evidence, for example, that lonely children are more likely to fall victim to sexual abuse and that predators know this (Rufo, 2012).

It is also important to keep in mind that not all traumatic events are equally pathogenic. Thus, for example, whereas childhood sexual abuse is an adversity that is often the most serious risk factor for many mental disorders, it does not reliably predict psychopathology in longitudinal follow-ups of children into adulthood (Fergusson & Mullen, 1999). My own research group (Paris et al., 1994a, 1994b) has examined the various parameters of abuse in BPD (relationship to perpetrator, duration, nature of the act, etc.) and found that long-lasting abuse from a caretaker or a partner of a caretaker had the most impact. Single incidents had less of an impact, especially if they did not involve physical contact. Finally, sexual abuse by an intimate partner during adolescence, however hurtful, did not by itself predict the development of BPD.

Why has the link between childhood trauma and BPD had such a strong hold on clinicians? First and foremost, it is a simple theory that tells a moving tale. (The long-term effects of trauma during childhood have been a theme in a large number of novels and films.)

Second, because most clinical patients of BPD are women, a traumatic model could be seen as consistent with a feminist perspective. This carries the danger that male clinicians who have a different view can be seen as failing to understand the challenges faced by woman in the modern world. As a therapist who has devoted so much of my career to treating women, I find that point of view unfair. For one thing, seeing women as victims, rather than helping them to become agents of their own destiny, goes against the principles of psychotherapy for either males or females. Accepting that there are heritable components in BPD in the form of personality traits need not be seen as invalidating life experiences.

Third, a trauma-focused model of BPD may be seen as consistent with a hope of prevention. However, treatment in mental health practice is now expected to be evidence based, and there are little or no data that demonstrate that prevention of major mental disorders, including BPD, is possible. We need to be more humble concerning what we know and what we do not know.

Fourth, the word "trauma" is a shorthand term that has been used to describe childhood adversities of all kinds (including neglect). We need to focus on a more subtle and pervasive role of family environment, a process that affects children over many years. All of us who are, or have been, parents know how long it takes to teach children emotional control. But when families dismiss or ignore problems in highly emotional children they are creating an environment that has been rightly described as invalidating.

We need to distinguish life events that are clearly traumatic (e.g., child abuse) from those that reflect an absence of proper care. The consequence of invalidation is that negative emotions are kept inside until they explode, so almost any rejection or disappointment can become a trigger for dysregulation.

The most common adversities reported by BPD patients (especially emotional neglect, i.e., a failure to provide support for upset feelings), as well as emotional abuse (criticism and devaluation) are forms of invalidation that fail to teach children how to handle their emotions. Again, these risks are much more common than highly traumatic events such as sexual abuse or family violence (Porter et al., 2020). Such risks can be dramatic but are reported by only about one-third of BPD patients (Yuan et al., 2023). If you insist on describing all form of child mistreatment as traumatic, I need to disagree. The present use of this term is misleading if it leads, as in Hollywood movies, to a search for single events that have catapulted patients into the realm of psychopathology.

The best data support the biosocial theory-based dialectical behavior therapy (Linehan, 1993). According to this model, BPD is related to emotion dysregulation, and emotion dysregulation is based on interactions between temperament (more intense emotions) and problematic responses by caretakers (invalidation).

Emotionality can be pathological when it is extreme. Failures of parenting are most damaging for those who are temperamentally vulnerable. Many people have strong reactions to their environment but do not develop psychopathology, largely because they have internalized a level of support from their families and significant others that keeps feelings from going out of control. They will be emotional and high-strung, but not disordered.

But when families dismiss or ignore problems in highly emotional children, that corresponds to an invalidating environment and leads to bad outcomes. The result is that negative emotions in children are kept inside until they explode and that almost any rejection or disappointment leads to dysregulation. Most patients with BPD report that they were misunderstood and that emotions were either ignored or dismissed. Telling a highly emotional person to snap out of it, or to grin and bear it, is not helpful and is a form of invalidation.

## SOCIAL RISK FACTORS IN BPD

Social factors can affect the risk of developing many forms of psycho-pathology. The main support for this conclusion is research showing that mental disorders can be more common in some social environments than they are in others (Paris, 2020b). Notable examples include eating disorders, substance abuse, and PDs. Eating disorders are partly related to the demands of modern society to have some degree of physical perfection. Substance use is more universal across cultures, but it is rare in societies that have controlled this kind of behavior in the form of social norms and structures that suppress impulsive behaviors of all kinds. For example, researchers decades ago found it hard to find any cases of antisocial personality disorder in the highly regulated traditional societies of Taiwan (Compton et al., 1991).

I have long been interested in whether BPD can be found in traditional societies (Paris & Lis, 2013). Almost 60 years ago, when I lived in India for nearly 2 years, I never heard anything about patients with the clinical features of BPD. Since then, times have changed, and underdeveloped countries have modernized. When I went back to visit this vast country decades later, mental health clinicians, especially in larger cities, were familiar with BPD.

The evidence that BPD has increased in prevalence in developed countries is indirect, largely because formal epidemiological studies of PDs have, until recently, been rather rare. But there have been notable increases in the frequency of certain symptoms during adolescence and youth that can be features of BPD, in particular suicidality, self-harm, and substance use.

Although the evidence is not strong enough to easily explain these changes, one hypothesis concerns the development of identity in an individualistic modern society (Kitayama et al., 2020; Paris, 2020b). People who grow up in traditional societies live by cultural norms and do not have to find their own identity, but in modern societies high levels of individuation are required. This demand on adolescents to find themselves is not a problem for everyone. Many who embrace the freedom to choose who they want to be in life benefit from modernity. But these trends tend to leave some people at biological and psychological risk without the social structures that can protect them against many forms of psychopathology.

In the process of finding a direction in life, young people are at greater risk of losing their way. A search for identity is hardly a new observation, but it underlies many of the symptoms of PDs.

## CLINICAL IMPLICATIONS OF THE BPS MODEL

The BPS model can also be a useful guide to therapy. In severe mental disorders, a strong biological predisposition is consistent with a focus on the treatment of patients with medication, but in BPD, even though it has a heritable component, pharmacological interventions are generally not useful. For example, antidepressants, which are prescribed routinely to patients with BPD, are rarely of great help, and they are not recommended by authorities such as Cochrane (Binks et al., 2006; Stoffers-Winterling et al., 2020). Antipsychotic drugs can sometimes reduce emotion dysregulation and impulsivity, but they do not lead to a remission of BPD itself, and they can have serious side effects if taken over long periods. Mood stabilizers are misnamed, because they are anticonvulsive drugs that only regulate mood swings in patients with bipolar disorders and are not of much value in BPD. (See Chapter 4 for further discussion of this issue.)

Unfortunately, many physicians who request consults on BPD patients prescribe heavily (sometimes up to five to six drugs), in the mistaken belief that they can separate depression or anxiety from BPD and treat these patients pharmacologically. This is a case where less is more. The fact is that medication adds little to outcome and leads to problematic polypharmacy that is not evidence based.

This conclusion emerges from a large body of research on treatment (Stoffers-Winterling et al., 2022; Storebø et al., 2020). Moreover, psychological interventions can also change brain functioning (Barsaglini et al., 2014). It is possible that in the future we will have drugs that are fairly specific to BPD, but for now, because BPD patients gain little from pharmacotherapy, I am more likely to discontinue agents that have previously been prescribed than to add any new ones.

Psychotherapy is quite sufficient to manage most cases of BPD, but therapists do not need to ground themselves too deeply in a single theoretical position. As I argue in this book, the idea that trauma is of central importance leads to therapies that are all too narrow in scope. It may be a cliché by now, but reviewing the past has limited value in dealing with the present. Patients need skills much more than they need to understand a traumatic past. This is why the therapies for BPD that have the strongest evidence base focus on the present and on solving current problems.

The good news is that a vast body of research supports the primacy of specialized psychotherapies for BPD. However, it is important to remember that these patients are more sensitive to triggering life events. That is a biological vulnerability that might limit the power of therapy, but it does not—any more than following a diet or avoiding substance use is an obstacle to medical treatment. The whole point of therapy for PDs is to modify traits that are not working for patients.

CASE EXAMPLE 3.1
## BIOPSYCHOSOCIAL RISK FACTORS IN BPD, I

Kaitlyn was a 26-year-old single woman on leave from a job as an administrative assistant in a hospital. Her most current problem was substance use, with up to 3g a day of cannabis, but also including frequent use of cocaine and the occasional use of psychedelics. Her problems with substances began in adolescence, when she became attached to peers who were also users, but they became more severe over time. Kaitlyn had been a cutter in her teens and had recently been seen several times in the emergency room after threatening suicide at the end of toxic relationships with men.

Kaitlyn's father was a serious alcoholic who was emotionally abusive, and he left the family when Kaitlyn was 5 years old. She was then raised by her mother, who was chronically depressed and unsupportive of emotional problems in her children. Kaitlyn was also a child of poverty who had to grow up in a high-crime neighborhood. She had never learned to manage emotions, only to survive exposure to multiple psychosocial risks.

CASE EXAMPLE 3.2
## BIOPSYCHOSOCIAL RISK FACTORS IN BPD, II

Leila was a 24-year-old single woman who had returned to university after first dropping out and then worked for several years in minimum-wage jobs. She had a history of self-harm and suicidality dating back to her early teens. She has had serious problems with addiction, and her father had been a drug dealer in the past. Leila's birth was unplanned, and her parents were both emotionally and physically neglectful. As a younger child, she benefited from the structure of primary school and living in a closely knit ethnic neighborhood. However, beginning in her early teens, Leila lacked the skills to regulate emotions, becoming a heavy drinker, and she has had violent quarrels with partners after which the police were several times called by neighbors.

CASE EXAMPLE 3.3

**BIOPSYCHOSOCIAL RISK FACTORS IN BPD, III**

Maya was a 22-year-old woman living with a male partner. After an argument with this partner, she took a large overdose and was unconscious for several hours. Maya's parents were immigrants from a developing country, and Maya had arrived in the country as a small child. The family struggled to adapt to their new life, and the parents, who were now running a restaurant, were rarely at home. Maya was a sensitive child with a volatile temperament. Her parents lacked the time or the inclination to validate and soothe her feelings. But when she entered the world of romantic relationships, she lacked the ability to communicate effectively about emotions, or to regulate them.

These three cases reflect the complexity of developmental psychopathology over time and the role of multiple interacting risk factors. In each of these cases, the patient faces biological risks (problematic temperament and a family history of a mental disorder), psychological risks (emotional neglect), and social risks (poverty and immigration). Each of these factors added to an overall burden of risk while interacting with each other in vicious cycles. In each of these cases, psychopathology emerged in the adolescent years, interfering with the mastery of tasks and skills that could have been invested in preparing a career and finding a social role. The complexity of the pathways to BPD in adolescence and youth requires a complex theoretical model.

## SUMMARY POINTS

- Mental disorders are best understood in a BPS model, and BPD is no exception.

- Biological risk factors in BPD are heritable and affect vulnerability to the environment.

- Psychosocial risk factors in BPD interact with this vulnerability in leading to the development of a mental disorder.

- BPD most often emerges in adolescence, which is a time when all these risk factors are more likely to be present.

PART **II** TREATMENT

# 4
# TREATMENT METHODS

In this chapter, I review evidence-based therapies that have been shown to be useful in treating borderline personality disorder (BPD). The best studied is dialectical behavior therapy (DBT), but all approaches capitalize on common factors in therapy: helping patients regulate emotions, reduce impulsivity, and improve interpersonal skills. This combination of the general and the specific is the basis of successful treatment regardless of the acronym used to describe it. In this chapter, I also explain why medications are usually not effective for BPD.

## SPECIFIC AND NONSPECIFIC FACTORS IN PSYCHOTHERAPY

The form of treatment for BPD that has the strongest evidence base consists of specialized forms of psychotherapy designed to address the key features of this disorder. Some are specific, and others are more nonspecific. But in each case, psychotherapy uses a therapeutic relationship to address symptoms related to emotion dysregulation and to teach skills that can modify the problematic traits that drive emotion dysregulation. These mainly include methods

https://doi.org/10.1037/0000440-005
*A Concise Guide to Borderline Personality Disorder*, by J. Paris

to increase emotion regulation through better distress tolerance and to reduce impulsivity by the early identification of emotions and learning how to control these feelings, as well as by learning better ways of managing relationships.

Let us begin by summarizing the overall mechanisms behind psychological treatment of any kind. As shown by many meta-analyses, psychotherapy works for most patients most of the time (Barkham et al., 2021). However, several limitations of this research need to be kept in mind. First, there is little evidence for specificity in psychotherapies in relation to outcome. Comparative trials of different methods have almost always found that therapies identified by brand names or acronyms are not superior to each other (Wampold & Imel, 2015). On the contrary, research suggests that the effectiveness of most therapies depends on common factors, such as a strong therapeutic alliance and a focus on problem solving. Thus, the current proliferation of so many different methods of psychotherapy is not supported by research (Barkham et al., 2021). Instead, evidence-based therapies with a defined structure and plan usually yield better results than what has been called *treatment as usual* (TAU), that is, the normal follow-up offered in most clinics. There are some exceptions: Addictions, eating disorders, and personality disorders (PDs) may require more specific methods and specialized interventions.

The importance of nonspecific factors in psychotherapy outcome has been known for decades, yet new therapies continue to be developed and are marketed to clinicians as unique. Yet the most consistent drivers of success are common factors. By and large, therapy works best when empathy is strong, when treatment focuses on current problems, and when therapists teach patients skills to manage these problems.

So, why are there so many psychotherapies, each with a different name? There are now hundreds of them, competing in a very crowded market, and often identified by three- or four-letter acronyms. However, treatments based on different theories and methods yield almost identical outcomes in head-to-head comparisons. The answer lies, once again, in the common factors that drive effective therapy (Wampold & Imel, 2015).

One of the problems in psychotherapy practice concerns the length of treatment. The perception that psychotherapy has to be long, expensive, or even interminable has been hard to remove. I have met patients who have been in therapy with multiple clinicians for most of their lives, yet research shows that most therapy in practice is brief (Stulz et al., 2013), and there is little evidence for treatment that continues for more than 1 year. One meta-analysis failed to show any advantage for longer over brief therapy

(Juul, Jakobsen, Jørgensen, et al., 2023). Moreover, all the evidence for the efficacy of psychotherapy of any kind is based on treatment lasting for a few months, or at most a year. We cannot say that continuing for longer than that makes any difference. Also, long therapies have a point of diminishing returns.

All of these findings suggest that psychotherapy is most effective when it is time limited and targeted. We should also be promoting therapies that are cost-effective (Lazar, 2010). Cost savings almost always emerge in practice, largely because treatment reduces unemployment and absences from work. For this reason alone, making evidence-based therapy accessible for a wider range of disorders should be a priority of mental health systems. As I argue in Chapter 5, we have a responsibility to make treatment more available.

Therapy for BPD is generally expensive and uses a lot of human resources, yet an Australian study in a public system confirmed that psychotherapy for BPD is actually cost-effective, saving the mental health system large amounts compared with TAU (Meuldijk et al., 2017). Although even TAU has some benefit in BPD (Finch et al., 2019), it does not compare to the outcomes from more specific therapies.

Moreover, psychotherapy usually works rapidly. For this reason, most patients, even those who have BPD, can be effectively treated for a few months (Paris, 2017). Our clinic manages most patients in this way (Laporte et al., 2018). Although some researchers have claimed that longer therapies are needed for complex disorders (Leichsenring et al., 2023), the evidence for that conclusion is weak. Without control groups and longitudinal follow-ups, research cannot support the idea that treatment works better than naturalized recovery over longer periods of time. Finally, only a few studies have compared shorter therapies with longer ones for BPD, and those that did have reported few differences (McMain et al., 2017). The use of open-ended therapies with no time limit also departs from the domain of evidence-based practice because it lacks support from clinical trials. Moreover, setting a time limit concentrates patient motivation and encourages behavioral change.

I am not claiming that all the problems associated with a BPD diagnosis can go away entirely after treatment that lasts a few months, but to meet the demand for treatment of this disorder therapists can be satisfied with whatever level of improvement can be achieved in a shorter time frame. Moreover, clinicians can assume patients can use what they have learned and remain on a trajectory of recovery, eventually graduating to the point that they become their own therapists, so to speak. Once patients take on that task, they can use the agency that comes from solving problems, and they do so without consulting a professional. When that does not happen, a second course of brief therapy may be needed, but that option is required for only a minority of patients.

In addition, although psychotherapies of all kinds remain the main form of treatment (Cristea et al., 2017; Crotty et al., 2024), no single method has been found to be superior to any other (Setkowski et al., 2023). Most of this evidence concerns DBT, but its superiority to alternative methods has not been established (Stoffers-Winterling et al., 2022).

Our program mainly uses the principles of DBT, but it is open to therapists trained in other traditions. We have built this consensus on the basis of decades of working together as a team. We do not offer a manualized guide to treatment but instead use a general framework that allows therapists to make use of their own training, experience, and comfort with different methods. Thus, although we spend more time on DBT skills, we leave room for psychodynamic work on adverse early experiences, for cognitive therapy emphasizing processing of life experiences, and for methods that focusing on mentalization (i.e., learning how to understand one's own mental state of oneself and the mental states of other people; Bateman & Fonagy, 2004). Thus, we use an eclectic mix of interventions and are not that concerned about individual differences in therapist style.

This having been said, because BPD is a complex disorder, standard methods (e.g., classical cognitive behavior therapy [CBT] or psychodynamic therapies) need to be modified. Although CBT designed for these patients also has some evidence for efficacy (Davidson et al., 2006), DBT, though based in part on CBT, uses a mix of other interventions. Psychodynamic treatment, once the most common option, now mainly takes the form of transference-focused psychotherapy (TFP), which has earned some evidential support for superiority to TAU (Doering et al., 2010).

The construct of BPD was originally developed by therapists looking for ways to treat patients who did not respond to ordinary methods. Linehan (2014a, 2014b) had a similar rationale for creating DBT, which is guided by an eclectic range of skills that can be taught to patients. Because BPD patients need structure, therapy needs to be quite active. BPD patients need advice that is based on the skills they can learn, as well as about what not to do. (It may be easier to make contracts with patients to control impulsivity than to teach them how to do things they have long been avoiding.)

It follows that therapies should not focus too much on the past at the expense of addressing current problems. Thus, when therapists understand that childhood trauma is not the main cause of BPD they can validate life histories without adopting models that are trauma focused. Even when trauma interferes with development, Linehan (1993) advocated moving on from a past that cannot be changed, introducing they key concept of *radical acceptance*. Where our clinic differs from the DBT model is that we do not impose a trauma focus that runs the risk of making treatment go on too long. Any therapy that lacks a time frame runs the risk of being endless as well as endlessly unproductive.

Although every therapist can have a unique perspective, not all will have read the research literature, and few have ever participated in or conducted clinical trials. Managing BPD is different from treating depression or anxiety because effective treatment involves interventions that focus less on symptoms and more on problematic personality traits, teaching patients how to regulate emotions, control impulsivity, and manage relationships. All evidence-based treatments keep these goals in mind.

## DBT

In the past, there was little reason to conclude that BPD patients were treatable. Clinicians often avoided these cases or tended to give them a different diagnosis that seemed more optimistic. The teachers who encouraged me to work with this population were untouched by a knowledge of research data. Decades ago, I invited a series of experts on BPD to my hospital to describe their methods with this population. They all spoke with eloquence, but only a few had ever conducted formal research to demonstrate either effectiveness or efficacy. Then, 30-odd years ago, there was finally a breakthrough.

DBT was the first method of treating BPD to gain support from randomized clinical trials (RCTs). Linehan et al. (1991) showed that DBT worked better than TAU. Linehan (1993) went on to write a widely read book describing her theory and clinical methods in some detail. Since then, at least 10 RCTs have supported the efficacy of DBT for BPD patients (Bedics, 2020; Stoffers-Winterling et al., 2022). Moreover, other disorders that have emotion dysregulation as a prominent symptom may also benefit from DBT (Cludius et al., 2020).

The uniqueness of DBT is that although it acknowledges the importance of life histories and early adversities, it applies guidelines on how to teach patient skills—in handling emotions, impulsive behaviors, and close relationships. Its methods are mainly aimed at teaching patients how to regulate dysregulated emotions. Countering emotion dysregulation involves identifying emotions, tolerating them, and finding better ways to get them under control. As noted, DBT is an eclectic mix of interventions, but it uses mindfulness skills that have been applied in several other forms of therapy. The difference between CBT and DBT is that DBT is a multimodal treatment that makes use of a broader range of interventions.

Decades after its introduction, DBT remains the most widely used model for treating BPD. Its structure includes both individual and group therapy, brief phone consultations with patients in crises, and regular consultations with colleagues for therapists. DBT has not been found to be superior to competing methods. It has not been found to be superior to a structured form of clinical management (McMain et al., 2009). As we will see, this comparison treatment, based on clinical guidelines, was later turned into another form of therapy. This lack of unique effects often emerges from research that compares DBT with other well-structured treatments. That is why researchers at the Cochrane policy institute have concluded that several kinds of psychotherapy of have reasonably good evidence (Stoffers-Winterling et al., 2022), but they do not specifically recommend DBT. Nonetheless, this method was a breakthrough, and every clinician who treats BPD needs to understand its theory and methods.

In some ways, DBT sets its goals too high. We know that this method is good at removing symptoms, but Linehan (1993) also proposed (in the absence of data) that to modify personality, several years of treatment might be needed. Until now, no research has studied longer term DBT. The outcomes of the clinical trials that support it depend mainly on finding that 1 year of treatment leads to reductions in suicidal and self-harm behaviors.

DBT remains the most researched method of treatment for BPD, but it is resource intensive, expensive, and difficult to access. In a public system, it requires the availability of skilled therapists with the support of hospitals and/or universities. Moreover, its length means that DBT clinics always have a significant wait list. Even in a private system, in which patients can afford to pay for treatment, people may need to wait for 6 to 12 months before they can begin DBT.

This means that DBT cannot usually be offered rapidly for crises. The year of treatment (the length that has been tested in clinical trials) includes weekly group therapy, individual therapy, and phone coaching. But the result is that a DBT program can cost tens of thousands of dollars over 12 months—well beyond the means of most patients, who usually lack good insurance (Brettschneider et al., 2014). The problem is even greater if one assumes that 1 year of treatment is just the beginning of a longer course. Yet there is no empirical evidence that DBT needs to last for more than 1 year. Again, note that randomized comparison of 12 versus 6 months of treatment at a university-based clinic in Canada yielded identical outcomes for both options (McMain et al., 2017). The authors of that study commented that sticking to a time limit was useful in mobilizing change.

There are also programs that offer therapy based on DBT principles but lasts for only a few months, aiming mainly to get symptoms under control. Others increase accessibility by offering group therapy only. These options are discussed in Chapter 5.

DBT has also been adapted for adolescents, the stage at which BPD usually begins to present. Evidence from clinical trials (Asarnow et al., 2021) as well as meta-analyses (Kothgassner et al., 2021) support its use for help with emotion dysregulation, self-harm, and suicidality in that population. One question is whether most adolescents with BPD are ready for therapy and will attend sessions regularly. For those who are ready, programs for this population are available. Alternatively, adolescents can be followed less systematically at that stage of life until they are ready to fully commit to treatment (Chanen et al., 2020).

## OTHER EVIDENCE-BASED THERAPIES

Let us now consider other methods for the treatment of BPD. I will restrict this discussion to those methods that have been tested in RCTs of their own; however, their research support is not as extensive as that for DBT.

### Mentalization-Based Treatment

Mentalization-based treatment (MBT) was developed by two psychoanalyst–researchers in the United Kingdom (Bateman & Fonagy, 2004, 2006). It offers a year or two of individual and group therapy. Its main idea is to teach patients how to *mentalize*, that is, to understand emotions in other people and in themselves. There is an overlap between the concept of mentalization and the mindfulness-related skills taught in DBT.

MBT is the only method of treatment for BPD that been examined in long-term follow-up studies to determine the stability of improvement after therapy. In contrast, DBT patients have been followed up for only 1 year after discharge (Linehan et al., 1993). But two studies, one on MBT in a day hospital setting (Bateman & Fonagy, 1999) and one in an outpatient clinic (Bateman & Fonagy, 2009), contacted patients after 8 years (Bateman et al., 2021; Bateman & Fonagy, 2008). The results indicated that MBT produces outcomes that remain stable over time.

Only one study has directly compared MBT with DBT (Barnicot & Crawford, 2019). It found that their outcomes were very similar. Although there were fewer dropouts in the MBT group, the choice of therapies was self-selected rather than randomized, and patients who chose DBT were more impaired at baseline. Also, the studies that support MBT have been conducted in the clinic where it was developed, and other groups have found few differences between it and standard therapy (Carlyle et al., 2020; Jørgensen et al., 2013).

MBT introduced several useful ideas, and because mentalization is a skill that can be taught it is compatible with programs that are based on DBT. However, MBT shares with DBT the limitation of being lengthy and expensive, making it less than widely accessible outside of the public sector.

## TFP

TFP is based on the theories of Otto Kernberg (Yeomans et al., 2002). It has thus far been supported by one RCT that compared it with TAU (Doering et al., 2010). The treatment offers weekly individual therapy, but not group therapy. As its name implies, TFP focuses on how patients replay interpersonal problems with their therapists, using that setting to teach better management of relationships. However, research has not proven that focusing on transference is a necessary part of this treatment.

## Schema Therapy

Schema therapy, developed by a cognitive therapist (Young, 1999), is an adaptation of CBT that focuses on how patients apply maladaptive schemas to current life problems. Its methods overlap the domains of cognition and psychodynamics. It has been less researched than other methods, with the most quoted trial finding it to be equivalent in outcome to TFP (Giesen-Bloo et al., 2006).

## General Psychiatric Management

General Psychiatric Management (GPM; Choi-Kain et al., 2016) was originally a comparison treatment based on clinical practice guidelines. It was found in a large-scale study to be equal in efficacy to DBT (McMain et al., 2009). GPM is general in the sense of its eclecticism; it applies ideas from several other methods. GPM was designed for office practices in which case management is the focus and when patients are seen individually on a weekly basis for up to 18 months. The method has been adapted for adolescents, known as *GPM-A* (Choi-Kain & Sharp, 2012). GPM uses many of the same strategies as DBT to deal with emotion dysregulation, and it can be offered in a stepped care model (Sonley & Choi-Kain, 2021). Patients are seen only once a week, but treatment can still be expensive if it lasts a full year.

### Other Evidence-Based Therapies

Some evidence-based therapies have offered group therapy alone, either by itself or as an add-on to individual follow-up. The most researched version of that approach is Systems Training for Emotional Predictability and Problem Solving (STEPPS; Blum et al., 2008; Van Wel et al., 2006). It offers individual and group therapy as a short-term package in settings where extended therapies are not available and is discussed further in Chapter 5 of this volume.

Livesley (2017) has written about a method that he calls "Integrated Modular Treatment," which also integrates multiple paradigms. This therapy does not set any time limit and may be adapted for open-ended therapy, in particular in Canada, where psychiatrists (but not psychologists) are insured by the government. It has not thus far been studied in clinical trials.

Again, although psychotherapy is the main treatment for BPD, none of the methods I have discussed so far seems superior to their competitors. Livesley (2012) offered a useful critique of all acronym-based therapies for BPD. He pointed out that because patients meeting criteria for this diagnosis are heterogeneous, each method approaches the problem from a different perspective without taking into account the full range of psychopathology in the disorder.

The most general conclusion I can draw from the research is that several methods of psychotherapy are successful in treating BPD patients. DBT remains the best researched option, but it has not been shown to be superior to other methods.

## HOW DOES PSYCHOTHERAPY HELP BPD PATIENTS?

Psychotherapists can be attracted to theories and methods that claim to be unique and definitive. All current therapies for BPD make such claims, and several are labeled with easily remembered acronyms. The developers of these treatments promote their approaches through conferences, workshops, journal articles, and books.

An integration of all methods, using their best ideas, has the potential to avoid unnecessary competition. In practice, all therapies for BPD have much in common and, as we have seen, comparative trials often find few differences in outcome between methods, in particular when the comparison is between specific methods and structured management rather than with TAU (Weinberg et al., 2011), yet allegiance to specific methods remains strong, even among researchers whose own studies do not necessarily support unique effects. The evidence continues to support the view that the various psychotherapies for BPD, however different their theories, tend to converge in practice. Let us therefore examine what all evidence-based treatments for BPD have in common.

### Emotion Dysregulation

This psychological construct, derived from research on emotions (Gross, 2014), has also been termed *affective instability* (Koenigsberg, 2010). It presents clinically as rapid changes in mood, often with rages, and is sometimes confused with bipolarity, but these mood swings last for hours, not for weeks.

Emotion dysregulation is central in the treatment of BPD. Stabilizing and processing these responses is a crucial element of all successful therapy. DBT took the lead (Linehan, 1993) by teaching specific skills. This method uses, for example, mindfulness, which is a central element of many cognitive therapies (Segal et al., 2002). Derived from Buddhist spiritual practices, mindfulness allows people to observe their thoughts calmly without acting on emotions. MBT also promotes emotion regulation by teaching patients to make accurate assessments of emotional states in interpersonal encounters. STEPPS is very similar in that patients are asked to chart their emotional states to monitor and control them. MBT and TFP, by asking patients to correct distorted perceptions, also promote self-observation.

### Behavioral and Interpersonal Skills

One of the most essential elements in all psychotherapies involves teaching patients better ways of managing interpersonal relations. Therapists can also encourage patients to deal with stress more productively, finding alternatives to cutting, overdosing, or abusing substances. Skills training in DBT covers a lot of ground and has been manualized (Linehan, 2014a, 2014b). MBT teaches patients to observe the subtleties of interpersonal relations, and STEPPS has modules for relationship skills. TFP implicitly teaches skills by pointing out how interpersonal problems also occur within a therapeutic relationship.

Therapies for BPD diverge in relation to technical procedures, which may or may not make a unique contribution to outcome. One example is the use of telephone coaching in DBT. In this model, therapists carry a pager to be available by phone to coach patients, who are encouraged to call when feeling emotionally dysregulated and about to carry out some form of self-harm. However, patients have to wait for a return call after leaving a message on a machine, and if they have already self-harmed, they may not get a call back.

Carrying a pager is a burdensome expectation for therapists, whose work is demanding enough as it is. We all need to protect our outside life to recharge our psyche. Most of us have families of our own and do not want to compromise precious time assigned to our personal lives. I understand that these contacts are brief and intended to reinforce skills, but when patients are already being seen twice a week, we can encourage them to practice tolerating a wait.

Moreover, there is no evidence that contact outside scheduled sessions makes a difference in outcome, given that the procedure is embedded in a wide-ranging treatment package. Only a dismantling strategy (Wampold & Imel, 2015), in which each intervention is removed to see which one really works, could determine which components of DBT are necessary and which are dispensable. DBT is a very complex treatment, so adapting it for brief therapy and broader use requires making choices.

Another example of differences between methods of therapies concerns the amount of time and attention one gives to exploring childhood events. This has always been a central difference between CBT and psychodynamic therapy, but although early adversities are common in BPD patients there are disadvantages in focusing on the past in patients who have so many problems in the present. Therapists should always validate painful feelings about the past but need not necessarily make them their main focus. Radical acceptance, avoiding a focus on the past, is, in my view, one of the most crucial ideas in DBT.

There is little evidence that specific techniques make a large difference in treatment outcome in BPD patients. Comparative trials do not demonstrate differences, in particular when both use structured methods. Thus, research has not supported the idea that technical procedures or theoretical principles lead to specific therapeutic effects; instead, patients benefit from coherent and well-structured methods that can involve different techniques and theories (Choi-Kain et al., 2016). Attachment to a single approach may prevent therapists from taking unique characteristics of patients into account (Livesley, 2017).

We need to take the absence of evidence for specific or brand names of therapy seriously. Clinical practice guidelines for BPD all concur that psychotherapy is the most effective treatment, but if they do not support one approach over others then therapists need not sign up for additional training. They can continue what they are already doing with modifications that are based on what research supports. In other words, instead of following treatment manuals, therapists can develop a form of eclecticism that reflects their own experience and what makes them most comfortable.

## TREATING BPD IN LIGHT OF PSYCHOTHERAPY INTEGRATION

The movement for psychotherapy integration (Norcross & Goldfried, 2019) has long taken a skeptical view of the uniqueness of specific theories or methods. Integrated therapy is more consistent with what research shows about how it works, in that common factors play the most crucial role. Patients of all kinds do best when treatment is based on a clear conceptual model, when there is a strong working alliance, when therapists provide empathy and validation, and when the emphasis is on problem solving in the present. The most effective therapy would be one that optimizes all the useful ingredients of "named" therapies (Castonguay et al., 2015). This principle has been the focus of advocates of an integrated approach to the treatment of BPD (Choi-Kain et al., 2016; Livesley, 2017).

Developing a common factors model could be particularly important for the clinical challenges presented by BPD (Paris, 2015). It is time to avoid allegiances to acronym-based therapies and to develop a practical model that clinicians can use without undergoing extensive training. Doing so could also make BPD treatment more available.

Psychotherapy integration has been supported by the findings of comparative trials in common mental disorders, in which differences between methods are not usually found (Norcross & Goldfried, 2019), but it has not been applied consistently to the treatment of BPD. Weinberg et al. (2011) described some of the common factors that have been scored with a standardized measure. A clear treatment framework, attention to affect, a focus on treatment relationship, and an active therapist, as well as exploratory and change-oriented interventions, characterized all methods. This conclusion is consistent with the psychotherapy integration literature as a whole.

On the basis of a general theory of PD treatment, Livesley (2017) derived very similar general principles: establishing a basic frame, maintaining a collaborative treatment alliance, maintaining a consistent treatment process, building motivation for change, and promoting self-reflection. In BPD, there are also specific goals: ensuring safety; containing symptoms, emotions, and impulses; regulating and controlling emotions and impulses; changing maladaptive behavior and interpersonal patterns; and integrating a more adaptive self-structure. This is also the view of those who practice on the basis of GPM, which describes itself as a general (rather than a specific) method, or as an add-on rather than as a replacement to current practices (Choi-Kain et al., 2016).

An integrated model will share many features with evidence-based therapies such as DBT, and clinicians should be aware of what is unique in other methods. Again, I do not consider it necessary to have extensive training in a single model to manage BPD, and I would encourage therapists to integrate what research has supported with what they are already doing.

## PHARMACOLOGICAL INTERVENTIONS IN BPD

Many clinicians who see patients with BPD find that they are already taking multiple medications prescribed by psychiatrists or family physicians, yet the evidence for this practice is rather weak. Most patients with BPD can manage without medication. The main exception is when they need a drug to combat insomnia. Our clinics routinely recommend reducing dosage or stopping agents that have usually been tried before but that physicians have been reluctant to discontinue for fear of relapses.

Antidepressants are useful for patients with severe depression, but these drugs are being almost routinely prescribed for lowered mood of any kind. Moreover, research has failed to find that selective serotonin reuptake inhibitors (SSRIs) have much value in BPD (Binks et al., 2006; Stoffers-Winterling et al., 2020). The reason is that mood symptoms in this population are not the same as in patients who do not have a PD. BPD patients rarely have extended periods of severe depression, but they do experience highly unstable moods. At best, antidepressants have sedative effects that can lower anxiety.

Antipsychotic drugs (atypical agents such as quetiapine or aripiprazole) can be used to manage the brief psychotic episodes that are sometimes seen in BPD. They have calming effects that can help somewhat with emotion dysregulation and that can be used for insomnia when other agents fail. For this purpose, the dose should be kept low. Quetiapine is the only medication in this group that has been tested for efficacy in BPD in a large clinical trial (Black et al., 2014). However, because that study was sponsored by the pharmaceutical industry, and because the doses used were much higher than is usual, this report does not provide evidence for routine use. Moreover, quetiapine, like other atypical antipsychotics, has a problematic side effect, a metabolic syndrome that resembles prediabetes (Binks et al., 2006).

Other second-generation antipsychotics, such as risperidal and olanzapine, have the same problem with metabolic side effects. Aripiprazole is an antipsychotic that has fewer of these effects, but because research on using it for BPD remains preliminary, it has not been approved by the U.S. Food and Drug Administration for this purpose (Valdivieso-Jiménez et al., 2023).

Mood stabilizers are misleadingly named. These agents were originally developed to treat epilepsy, and they can stabilize mood in bipolar disorders, but they have little or no value for controlling the mood swings seen in BPD. The only large-scale effectiveness trial for one of these agents (lamotrigine) in BPD failed to find any effect at all (Crawford et al., 2018). Years later, I am amazed to see how few clinicians have read the article that reported this trial and how many still prescribe lamotrigine for BPD. This demonstrates, as in depression, how easily it is to be misguided by the name of a group of drugs.

Because of their problems with attention, many BPD patients today are being put on stimulants; however, that is not an evidence-based practice. Attention problems can also arise from emotion dysregulation, anxiety, depression, or interpersonal conflicts. Attention-deficit/hyperactivity disorder (ADHD) is currently being overdiagnosed in adults, even though many patients lack the childhood onset of ADHD required for diagnosis by the *Diagnostic and Statistical Manual of Mental Disorders* (5th ed., text rev.; American Psychiatric Association, 2022; Paris et al., 2015). Moreover, people without ADHD will also focus better with stimulants, just as they do with coffee or tea.

Benzodiazepines have long been used to control anxiety. They are occasionally useful on a short-term basis for insomnia (Binks et al., 2006), but some patients will become addicted to them. They should only be used with caution.

Overall, no medication is specific to BPD, and most options have placebo effects when first prescribed that do not last. The only drugs that have even a limited role in the management of BPD are low-dose antipsychotics, but they should not be routinely prescribed.

Cochrane reports have been consistently skeptical of published findings on pharmacotherapy for BPD (Storebø et al., 2020). By and large, antidepressants are ineffective, mainly because chronic depression and mood instability are not the same thing as a major depressive episode without a comorbid PD (see Chapter 1). This has not stopped physicians and psychiatrists from prescribing them, even if patients do not benefit or have only a short-term placebo response. And the fad for overdiagnosing ADHD means that many patients with PDs are also being prescribed stimulants, which have little evidence for their efficacy in BPD. There could, however, be a role for drugs that reduce the craving for substances and for nonsuicidal self-injury. Although there have been no clinical trials of the use of naltrexone in BPD (Del Casale et al., 2021), one may consider prescribing it when self-harm is severe.

My conclusion is that the majority of BPD patients can be managed without any form of medication. Moreover, once patients have been prescribed drugs, physicians tend to maintain them for years. And if one drug does not work, current medical practice favors adding another; it is not unusual to see BPD patients who are on four to five different medications. It could be said that physicians are better at adding than subtracting. But poly-pharmacy, in which patients are given multiple medications for years, is more likely to yield unpleasant side effects than a remission of BPD. For this reason, our programs spend more time taking patients off medications instead of increasing the side-effect burden. Psychiatrists have to know how to subtract as well as add.

CASE EXAMPLE 4.1
## PROBLEMS WITH POLYPHARMACY

Yasmine was a 24-year-old visual artist living with a boyfriend of 18 months. A previous psychiatrist had put her on a wide range of medications, including an SSRI, a benzodiazepine, an antipsychotic, and a stimulant.

The main work of her therapy focused on emotion regulation. Early on in therapy, as she learned skills for control of her emotions, Yasmine stopped self-harm (cutting). She then agreed to taper herself off all the meds, one by one. This process took a few months, and she had particular challenges in stopping the SSRI. However, once she felt she had achieved control of inner feelings, she was able to leave the program medication free.

This case illustrates the negative effects of polypharmacy, which reduces agency for patients while leaving them to cope with a heavy burden of side effects.

## TREATABILITY AND RECOVERY IN BPD

The evidence reviewed in this chapter shows that in spite of long-held clinical beliefs to the contrary, most patients with BPD can be successfully treated. However, a minority are either unsuitable for therapy and/or remain chronic and intractable. Because research on this subpopulation is thin, the information in this section is largely based on clinical experience.

A large empirical literature shows that patients with better psychosocial functioning prior to entering therapy are more likely to benefit from treatment (Barkham et al., 2021). In other words, people who work (or go to school to prepare for work), and who have meaningful relationships, do better than those who do not.

In the long run, however, work is more important than love. This is because a job provides a structure to daily life and a social role. I have treated patients from all walks of life over the years, from medical colleagues to cashiers in stores. Not every job is a meaningful career. But I always advise patients that work (or courses to prepare to work) is part of the treatment and that remaining unemployed undermines therapy. To be at home and collecting welfare is poison for most patients. It leads to social isolation, with the result that they lack a laboratory experience to test out any skills we are teaching. Moreover, if you do not have a job, you may look too much to relationships to fill your emptiness. This is why we insist that patients be either working or in school within the first few weeks of therapy. (Some programs in our area do not even allow patients to start until they meet that expectation.)

That is why love is a very different story. BPD is a disorder in which many of its symptoms develop in romantic relationships. These are patients who fall in love rapidly and who fall out of love almost as fast. They want too much from their partners and easily feel rejected, which makes intimacy a highly volatile experience. If patients are in a toxic relationship (and many are), we may gently advise them to consider leaving partners. And if, as often happens, they enter treatment just after a breakup, we advise them not to date until they feel better about themselves and can manage being alone. Love should not come before work in the lives of people with BPD (Choi-Kain et al., 2016). It asks too much of a partner, however good their intentions. You have to be somebody in order to love somebody properly.

With these guidelines in mind, what can we recommend for patients who are permanently unemployed, socially isolated, or both? Many have had BPD in the past but no longer meet diagnostic criteria. Some of these patients still seek therapy for emotion dysregulation. In such cases, expectations have to be lowered, and clinicians have to accept serious limitations. In this scenario, therapy resembles a rehabilitation process in which patients are asked to search for some sort of activity that is meaningful enough to be adopted and invested. This may be anything from volunteer work to hanging out with other people at a shopping mall.

Finally, some BPD patients are either not ready for specialized therapy or have comorbidities and personality traits that interfere with establishing a therapeutic alliance. An obvious example of a problematic comorbidity is serious drug or alcohol addiction. We tell these patients to get into rehabilitation programs and come back when they have been clean for 6 months. Then there are patients who have paranoid traits to the point where they trust almost no one, including a therapist. This trait may be slow to change if it has been present for most of a patient's life.

We are also careful about accepting patients with a serious forensic history, in particular if they are male. That is mainly because of our concern about protecting other people in group therapy with BPD patients, who are mainly female.

Some patients, adolescents in particular, can have symptoms are too "hot" for therapy and need to cool down first. Those who are too impulsive may not yet be ready to make a commitment to therapy. A related scenario relates to problems with frequent fliers to the emergency room—and these patients often fail to follow up in a crisis clinic. (Although we did successfully manage one patient who had been coming to the emergency room every day for several years.)

Keep in mind that a fair number of patients with BPD (over 20%) will drop out of psychotherapy (Iliakis et al., 2021). Some researchers have described even higher levels (Woodbridge et al., 2021), but that high a rate could occur in patients receiving TAU in community treatment rather than evidence-based therapies. We also have seen an approximate 20% dropout level in our own program. This problem, like much else in BPD, arises from dysregulation and impulsivity. Given the nature of this population, keeping a majority of the patients we see in therapy should be considered entirely acceptable. We are pleased that most patients stay with treatment and can be expected to benefit from it. We are also open to seeing patients again at a later point when they are more ready to make a commitment.

CASE EXAMPLE 4.2

## RESPONSE TO PSYCHOTHERAPY, I

Tania was a 24-year-old woman who came to our clinic after a hospitalization for an acute psychotic episode. She stayed in the program for two 6-month periods that were interrupted by a busy school schedule. Her symptoms included suicidality, residual paranoid ideas, and a history of choosing highly unsuitable romantic partners who mistreated her.

Tania was raised by a depressed single mother who never validated her emotions. Over the course of the treatment, she avoided having intimate relationships that she lacked the skills to manage. She benefited from the support of group therapy and the safety of individual therapy. By the end of treatment, she had a greater sense of identity and purpose, with suicide no longer an option. She still experienced paranoid ideas (e.g., the fear of someone coming to her house to kill her), but she was better able to dismiss these thoughts. As she progressed in her studies, she gained a better sense of direction in life and decided to postpone intimacy with men until she had an identity of her own.

---

**CASE EXAMPLE 4.3**
## RESPONSE TO PSYCHOTHERAPY, II

Sarah was a 28-year-old administrative assistant whose life centered around a sexually charged but volatile relationship with a boyfriend. Sarah was addicted to male attention and had been promiscuous in the past, but these problems ultimately reflected a lack of family support and validation. Over the past 3 years, Sarah had been entirely estranged from her parents, whom she felt understood her poorly or not at all. A brief course of therapy encouraged her to repair this loss of family, and she was able to lower her expectations, which allowed her to be eventually reunited with her parents.

---

These two case examples show how patients can recover from BPD through different pathways and how psychotherapy targeting emotion regulation, impulsivity, and dysfunctional relationships can guide them toward remission.

The evidence for the overall treatability of BPD is strong. This disorder benefits from a well-structured psychotherapy and does not necessarily require medication. However, one should not assume that any old therapy will do. (That is why TAU is used as a control condition in clinical trials.) If therapists have a well-thought-out plan and can draw on the personality issues that lie behind symptoms, they will usually be successful. The DBT model offers the clearest formulation of these issues, but there is no need to follow it slavishly or to ignore the contribution of other models.

It must also be acknowledged that some patients do not respond to even the most skilled therapy, but that is an issue for all the patients clinicians see. We can be (and should be) satisfied if most get better. As I discuss in the next chapter, only about 12% of our cases in brief treatment come back asking for more (Laporte et al., 2018).

Whether therapy is long or short, ending a course of formal treatment is only the beginning of a long process. Patients need to continue honing the skills needed to manage the expected (and unexpected) vicissitudes of life.

## SUMMARY POINTS

- There is strong evidence for the use of psychotherapy as the form of treatment that has the strongest evidence base for BPD, but specialized methods are needed to teach skills.

- The strongest evidence is for DBT, but it has not been established as being superior to other methods.

- An integrated model that combines the best ideas from multiple sources can be used.

- There is only weak evidence for the use of psychopharmacological agents in BPD.

# 5 ACCESS TO THERAPY FOR BORDERLINE PERSONALITY DISORDER

In this chapter, I review evidence that many, if not most, borderline personality disorder (BPD) patients can be effectively treated within a few months and do not necessarily require years of therapy. On the basis of a stepped care model, patients can be separated into groups that are most likely to benefit from brief interventions and those who need longer therapy.

## ACCESS TO TREATMENT FOR BPD PATIENTS

We know that most patients with BPD can benefit from treatment and that psychotherapy is the most effective option. Moreover, we can now choose from several evidence-based methods. That is the good news. The bad news, though, is that efficacious treatment is expensive and not readily available or accessible to those who most need it.

Many, if not most, current therapies are designed to last for a year or more, and some programs also ask patients to come twice a week for a combination of individual and group therapy. This lengthy time scale leads to problems with access to health care. The first problem is that the demand

https://doi.org/10.1037/0000440-006
*A Concise Guide to Borderline Personality Disorder*, by J. Paris

for therapy is always greater than the supply, so clinics offering treatment of any length inevitably develop waiting lists. Also, needless to say, waiting is a problem for patients with BPD. We need accessible treatments for crisis situations that do not leave patients on a wait list as well as therapies that can be accessed by a wider patient population.

The second problem is that the longer a therapy is, the greater will be its cost. In the United States, insurance for mental health treatments of all kinds is spotty (Lazar et al., 2018). Those who work for a large company or are military veterans will be better insured. Those who come from wealthy families may not even have this problem. But BPD is a condition that usually interferes with higher education and career trajectories, and few patients are able to accumulate sufficient savings to pay for a long course of mental health treatment. Even those who have insurance from work may be covered for only a few sessions. Few of the patients with BPD we see can afford a whole year of therapy. Even in Canada, which fully insures the work of physicians, the government does not cover psychologists (i.e., nonmedical providers) who work outside of hospitals. In most countries, including the United States, only a few specialized clinics for BPD exist in the public sector (Plakun & Villela, 2019).

Thus, although many patients with BPD have, in theory, effective specialized treatments at their disposal, most cannot readily access them. To address these problems, treatment needs to be offered in the public sector, either in outpatient settings or community clinics, and it needs to be shortened. Doing so would save money, if treatment leads to fewer visits to emergency rooms (ERs), a lower number of outpatients, or fewer admissions to the hospital (Lazar, 2010).

Most experts on BPD agree with the need for greater accessibility. Years ago, Zanarini (2009) wrote that "less intensive and less costly forms of treatment need to be developed" (p. 376). Similarly, McMain et al. (2012) recommended, "Given the lack of availability of effective treatments for BPD, research is needed on the effectiveness of less intensive models of care in order to help inform decisions about the allocation of scarce health care resources" (p. 650).

One problem is that too many patients are being seen for too long, blocking openings for others languishing on a wait list. In the absence of evidence, we should not assume that longer therapy is better. As I discussed in Chapter 4, there are no empirical data showing that therapy lasting longer than a year for any mental disorder is required, a principle that can be applied to BPD. Instead, a good deal of evidence shows that good results can be obtained in periods ranging from a few months to a year.

For example, a study from a large dialectical behavior therapy (DBT) clinic in Canada (McMain et al., 2022) found no difference in outcome between patients who were in therapy for 12 months (the length for which the treatment has been tested in clinical trials) and those in a course of therapy that lasted for 6 months. The authors suggested that a shorter option actually motivates patients to work harder at their treatment. Similar findings were reported in a comparison of mindfulness-based therapy over 5 months versus over 14 months (Juul, Jakobsen, Hestbaek, et al., 2023; Juul, Jakobsen, Jørgensen, et al., 2023). These findings support the view that if we can triage most cases we see in practice, and treat more of them briefly, we can reach more people struggling with BPD.

## EVIDENCE FOR BRIEF THERAPY IN BPD

We now know much more about how to treat BPD, yet we lack the resources to provide evidence-based care to many patients (Iliakis et al., 2019). This is why a number of treatment methods have been developed to provide brief and more accessible therapy. One meta-analysis supported a number of these short-term interventions (Spong et al., 2021). Research has shown that brief interventions reduce symptoms, most particularly emotion dysregulation, self-harm, and suicidality. And although some think that symptomatic improvement is not the same as personality change, giving up maladaptive behaviors also changes the way patients handle their interpersonal relationships.

Systems Training for Emotional Predictability and Problem Solving (STEPPS; Blum et al., 2008) applies a theory and methods similar to DBT in that it focuses mainly on emotion regulation skills. STEPPS does not provide individual therapy but is offered in groups over a period of 3 months. That is because the program was developed for patients who had other forms of follow-up (corresponding to treatment as usual) but had no access to therapy specific to BPD. This scenario makes STEPPS particularly suitable for settings outside large cities. Its efficacy has been supported by three clinical trials (Blum et al., 2008; Soler et al., 2009; Van Wel et al., 2006), as well as by an effectiveness study (Bos et al., 2011) and a systematic review (Ekiz et al., 2023).

Similarly, some clinical trials of DBT skills in groups limited to 20 sessions without individual therapy also have shown efficacy (McMain et al., 2017). Emotion regulation skills, a key element in DBT, have the same value in briefer therapy. In Switzerland, Kramer et al. (2020, 2022) have published data on a 10-session intervention. Although the authors described this brief intervention as intended as a "first step," it also makes therapy accessible. Similar methods have been described by other research groups (e.g., Sauer-Zavala et al., 2023). A protocol lasting for 12 weeks (Zanarini & Frankenburg, 2008) was also described as "pretreatment." However, there is no reason not to consider brief interventions as treatments, if they get patients on a trajectory of recovery that can continue after finishing therapy. It is not clear that most BPD patients will need a longer course. The majority do not, although an important minority does require more.

Thus, shorter therapy can be the key to better access. But the question we need to ask is this: Which patients are most likely to benefit from brief intervention, and which patients need a longer course (of up to a year)? Therapy that extends beyond 12 months is outside the domain of evidence-based practice.

## STEPPED CARE FOR BPD

Stepped care is designed for the treatment of disorders (medical and psychiatric) that have a variable prognosis. One triages patients by offering brief therapy to most cases while reserving more extensive and expensive treatment for those who do not or cannot complete the first step (or who have a severe disability). The principles of stepped care can be applied to BPD (Grenyer et al., 2018; Paris, 2013, 2017).

Our own clinic's stepped care program is based on many of the principles of DBT, but it makes use of ideas drawn from other models (Paris, 2022b). It offers most patients 11 weeks of individual and group therapy, and it offers extended care (6 or 12 months) for more chronic cases. Although we do not have data to support the value of this kind of triage, and although I have emphasized that the outcome of BPD is not very predictable, it fits our clinical experience. We started the program in 2002 by accepting everyone for brief therapy but changed our model after the first few years. The patients who come to our extended care program may no longer meet BPD criteria, but they retain emotion dysregulation, often while giving up on intimacy. In general, we offer extended care to two groups: (a) those who do not successfully complete the first step and come back later with continued distress and (b) those who are older and have more long-lasting and severe psychosocial dysfunction.

Data from a study my colleagues and I conducted (Laporte et al., 2018) show that the majority of patients in both programs can be treated successfully in a few months. Out of 479 patients we saw in the first 15 years of our program, only 60 (12%) came back asking for more therapy.

We now manage about 80 to 100 patients per year in the short-term program and about 30 to 40 in extended care. We have increased staffing from when we started, and now we can manage a larger number who ask for treatment. The original goal of this short-term program, located in a university hospital, was to make treatment available rapidly (usually within 2 months after assessment). However, we have been unable to avoid a wait list (many months) for patients who are referred to more extended care. The wait list for a 6- to 12-month course of therapy is much shorter (about 1 month) at most clinics in our network. In two other hospitals that limit availability to specific areas of our city, patients are seen for 6 months (with an option for 12), and the wait for programs is only 1 to 2 months. (In our province, access to mental health treatment is governed by sectorization, in which each hospital has a catchment area from which it draws its patients.) In contrast, our brief (11-week) program is located in a large hospital complex that covers all of Montreal and its suburbs.

When the short-term treatment program, founded in 2001, began, we took any patient referred to us. We quickly learned that brief treatment was most suitable for younger and actively symptomatic patients, who are the majority of patients seen in our clinics and ER. However, brief treatment was less effective for older patients who had not recovered from BPD. After the first few years, we triaged all referrals, sending the majority to a brief course of therapy while opening a separate clinic that offered extended care for this more chronic subpopulation.

When we started the clinic, our main aim was to relieve pressure on the ER by providing rapid access to therapy. We chose a length of 12 weeks (including a total of 24 sessions, with both weekly group and individual sessions) in accordance with established standards in cognitive behavior therapy (CBT). (We later reduced that length to 11 weeks in order to run four programs a year.)

Data on the first 15 years showed that most patients achieved significant reductions in symptoms and that the vast majority (88%) did not come back (Laporte et al., 2018). Because we are one of the largest facilities for BPD treatment in our city (as well as in Canada), when former patients present in other clinics and hospitals in our community they are routinely sent back to us. We are currently collecting formal follow-up data to ensure that improvements are stable over time.

We are not alone in proposing briefer therapy for BPD. Several other groups have found that 2 to 3 months of treatment has a significant effect on symptoms (see Spong et al.'s [2021] review). There is a stepped care program in Australia (Grenyer et al., 2018), but it treats most patients for 18 months. I doubt whether that length of therapy is necessary for most people with BPD.

Some of my colleagues have been incredulous that a severe mental disorder like BPD can be managed in less than a year, not to speak of several years. They were taught that long-term problems require long-term therapy, an idea that has long been a received wisdom guiding clinical practice. Our group does not claim that all patients with BPD can attain a full remission in a few months, only that the majority achieve a symptomatic remission and that these outcomes are meaningful and usually lasting.

Moreover, as I mentioned in Chapter 2, most BPD patients continue to recover over time without having longer courses of formal therapy. Follow-up studies, lasting as long as 24 years (Zanarini, 2019), have shown that once patients enter a trajectory of recovery they continue to improve, even without further therapy.

In the early years of our program we benefited from the support of a large hospital, in particular when clinicians noted that the burden on its emergency services eased after the clinic opened. We have been most successful with younger patients with acute symptoms such as emotion dysregulation, suicide attempts, self-harm, and dysfunctional relationships. These are the problems that bring patients to clinical attention (most often in an ER), but they also define a population that can have an early recovery. Focusing on younger patients was not a bias: BPD is a disorder that remits in most cases by age 30 to 40, and many are symptomatically recovered even earlier (Gunderson et al., 2003, 2011).

As noted, patients who are less likely to benefit from brief therapy have problematic comorbidities. Substance use (and eating disorders), when severe, often need to be managed first. When these problems take over patients' lives, we refer them to specialized clinics and accept them only once substance use is under better control. Our message for heavy users is "Get clean, then come back."

We also see patients with low levels of psychosocial functioning (e.g., chronic unemployment, lack of a social network) that make the prognosis of BPD doubtful. Our view, shared by many experts (Choi-Kain et al., 2016), is that patients who, for long periods, are not working or going to school to prepare for work are not yet treatable. There is little to talk about with patients who lack a life where they can test out learned skills. Our standard message in this case is "You need to get a job or go to school to prepare for one, or at least have a definite plan to do so, before entering treatment."

The need for a social role is why we give a higher priority to work than to love in patients with BPD. Many try to solve their problems through love, but that strategy will not succeed in the absence of a life that is meaningful in other ways. Without a social role, therapy will be like a science course that has lectures without a laboratory component. Patients need to be at work or school to practice skills related to emotion regulation and interpersonal relationships. Staying at home with little to do except for screen time is a recipe for treatment failure.

Our program is also asked to assess patients who have lifetime but not current BPD, as well as a smaller number who continue to meet full diagnostic criteria in middle age. This reflects a common trajectory of the disorder in a minority of cases. Some highly chronic patients go on long-term disability and stay there indefinitely. Others give up on having relationships, developing an avoidant pattern that protects them (i.e., not having intimacy because it is too difficult). This subpopulation can be referred to extended care, but we have not found that keeping these patients in therapy for longer than 1 year has any added benefit. The most common pattern in this type of patient is one of emotion dysregulation and mood swings in the absence of severe impulsivity or chaotic interpersonal relationships.

In a sense, all mental disorders lie on a spectrum of some kind, and BPD is no exception. As referrals to our clinic have steadily increased, we have had to turn down many cases, even though they may need treatment for other personality disorders (usually fitting only an "unspecified" category). This is because our primary mandate is to offer treatment to severely ill patients who need to be kept out of ERs.

With the increased recognition of personality disorders in the clinical community, our clinic is asked to evaluate patients who have some features of BPD but do not meet diagnostic criteria. For this group, we have one other option. One of the psychologists who worked with us for some years opened a private clinic offering 12 weeks of individual and group therapy at a lower rate than what is charged by most clinicians in private practice. In addition, some of the community clinics where therapists work that are funded by the Canadian government now offer short-term group therapy with a DBT focus.

Our program now treats more than 100 patients each year (80 short term and 30 in extended care). Since we started, we have managed the cases of several thousand people with BPD. Although the program has been supported by effectiveness data, we are planning to conduct controlled trials in the future to determine efficacy. However, we do not believe that the clinical improvements we have seen are placebo effects or examples of regression toward the mean. We consider that we are making the naturalistic recovery of BPD move significantly faster.

Our main difficulty at this point is that even with increased human resources, and while running the largest program in Canada, we are still not able to keep up with the demand for services. However, we can now rely on similar clinics at other hospitals in the McGill University network, as well as in a group of hospitals belonging to a French-speaking network associated with the University of Montreal. We are also pleased that social workers and psychologists in community clinics are now offering similar programs, all based on the principles of DBT, modified for short-term therapy.

A stepped care model offers brief therapy to most patients with BPD, but even in extended care all patients are encouraged to commit themselves to change within a specific time frame. We also see a smaller number of highly chronic and low-functioning patients who, because of the severity of their pathology, may not benefit from either program, especially group therapy. For this group, we run a smaller program that resembles treatment as usual, consisting of monthly follow-ups and focusing on support and medication management.

For most patients, whether treated for 11 weeks or 12 months, we offer both individual and group sessions. We consider group therapy, in which skills are taught, crucial for this patient population. Our experience is that the model we use, which is largely adapted from DBT, fits well the needs of younger patients with acute symptoms that bring them to ERs.

Our extended care clinic offers two kinds of group therapy, one focusing on skills and the other a classical process group. Individual therapy in both clinics combines DBT principles with an eclectic range of ideas drawn from other sources, including CBT, mindfulness-based therapy, and psychodynamic therapy, allowing us to take individual life histories into account. Groups allow us to teach emotion regulation and interpersonal skills in a supportive environment This combination of methods has been part of the most successful ways to treat BPD.

Commitment is an important expectation for all patients. We are very strict about attendance. We set a limit on the number of allowed absences for any reason: no more than two in an 11-week program and no more than six in a 6-month program. Those who cannot meet this expectation retain the option of returning at a later point and asking for more treatment. We find that these boundaries help keep motivated patients in treatment and keep unmotivated patients out until they are more ready. However, even in our extended care program, patients who are more chronic do not always do well. They will generally end up being followed in the community by physicians, psychologists, or social workers.

CASE EXAMPLE 5.1
## THERAPY IN 12 WEEKS

Thea was an 18-year-old woman attending a community college. When stressed by failed relationships, she would go into rages, and she sometimes heard voices in her head telling her she was a bad person.

Thea presented to the ER after an overdose. She had been self-harming since early adolescence. Substance use, mostly of cannabis, also became a problem, more so given that her parents were both alcoholics. With this in mind, and with the encouragement of the therapist, Thea stopped using cannabis in the first few weeks of therapy.

Thea was encouraged to continue with her studies, to concentrate on building a career plan, and to take a break from intimacy. Her strengths in college helped her to cooperate with the program. She also learned emotion regulation skills in group therapy, was discharged after 12 weeks, and did not come back for further follow-up.

This case is fairly typical of a successful brief therapy.

CASE EXAMPLE 5.2
## THERAPY IN 6 MONTHS

Angela was a 24-year-old woman seen for 6 months in our clinic. Her problems included difficult relationships with family and partners as well as a lack of close friends. Another important issue in her life was that her father, who sold drugs, eventually died in prison.

Angela had a problematic relationship with a man that ended because of his lack of commitment and support. She was encouraged to make female friends in order to avoid excessive emotional dependency on one man. She became less demanding of her mother, who never gave her what she needed, and she learned how to lower her expectations, and thus was better able to relate to her.

This case was somewhat more complex and therefore benefited from a 6-month course.

CASE EXAMPLE 5.3
## THERAPY IN 12 MONTHS

Belinda was a 31-year old woman with a career in business. She entered our clinic after an overdose that brought her to the ER. Many of her problems arose from a dysfunctional family in which her parents had paid little attention to her emotional needs. Most symptoms emerged in intimate relationships with men, but there were extensive periods during which she did not have relationships. Belinda had left her last partner because of his inability to calm her down whenever she was profoundly upset.

The focus of therapy was to validate Belinda's emotional needs and to counter an internalized feeling of being difficult and unlovable. In group therapy, Belinda learned skills that allowed her to regulate emotions, and she became less impulsive and dysfunctional in intimate relationships.

This case is an example of the more limited goals we set when we treat patients for as long as 12 months.

## EFFICACY, EFFECTIVENESS, AND COST-EFFECTIVENESS

Efficacy trials such as randomized clinical trials (RCTs) are considered the gold standard in medical and psychological treatment, but they have an important limitation in that patients who agree to be randomized may not be representative of the larger population with the same psychopathology. Effectiveness trials tell a different story. Although these data are limited by the absence of a control group, we need not assume that patients with BPD will improve within a short time without any treatment. Effectiveness data are useful because large and unselected clinical populations in which multiple comorbidities offer a better approximation of the larger population of BPD patients.

Several RCTs have measured the efficacy of psychotherapy in BPD, as summarized in Cochrane reports (Stoffers-Winterling et al., 2022; Storebø et al., 2020), and their conclusions have been supported by a large-scale meta-analysis (Cristea et al., 2017). RCTs help ensure that treatment effects are not just due to the treatment acting as a placebo. We were surprised at first to see how much better our own patients were after 12 weeks of treatment, but one of our founding therapists reminded us that evidence-based CBT traditionally lasts for about 20 sessions.

Most of our patients have had multiple visits to ERs with suicide threats or attempts, yet they can be taught how to be less dysregulated and impulsive. Most go back to work or school, put suicidality on hold, suspend impulsive behaviors, and learn to avoid choosing abusive partners. Although specialized programs for BPD patients cost money, they save much more. As discussed in Chapter 4, the main reason why is that when people go back to work or school they are no longer a drain on benefits provided by governments. Add to that savings due to reductions in demand for expensive interventions (e.g., medical workups) or psychiatric evaluations (often carried out in busy ERs). We are fortunate to be supported by generous insurance from the Canadian province where we work. In countries like the United States, insurance companies and government agencies need to know that BPD treatments are cost-effective. Making them accessible through better insurance calls for advocacy.

There is a larger role for advocacy by clinicians and researchers who work with and study patients with BPD. Zimmerman (2015) contrasted the level of advocacy for bipolar disorder with that for BPD. He concluded that researchers studying bipolar disorder have

> repeatedly demonstrated the economic costs and public health significance of bipolar disorder. In contrast, researchers of BPD have almost completely ignored each of these issues and thus have been less successful in highlighting the public health significance of the disorder. (p. 8)

The best way to bring clinicians around has been to demonstrate that BPD is treatable. And although we would like treatment to be more available than it currently is, many more clinicians are borderline-aware than they were 20 years ago.

## THE ROLE OF FAMILY SUPPORT

If you know anyone who is the parent of a child with BPD, you will already be aware that looking after someone who is deeply troubled and potentially suicidal is a huge challenge. Where can parents look for help?

The United States has an important organization, the National Education Alliance for Borderline Personality Disorder (NEA-BPD; https://www.borderlinepersonalitydisorder.org/), which was founded by a talented social worker, the late Perry Hoffman. Some years ago, the National Institute of Mental Health partnered with NEA-BPD to sponsor a series of conferences at various sites in the United States (as well as in Canada and the United Kingdom) to promote awareness of BPD as a public health problem and to educate people that it is a treatable disorder. Each of these meetings was cosponsored by organizations that educate and support families with a member who has BPD. I considered this initiative to be a success, and I am proud to have been part of it.

One of the most persuasive of advocates for the cause of access to care for BPD has been Valerie Porr, who has maintained a long-standing connection to the BPD research community. Valerie wrote an excellent book on BPD directed at families who have a member with BPD (Porr, 2010). She has also been active in lobbying the U.S. Congress for awareness of the disorder. Valerie also offers phone consultations to families across the United States about how to manage difficult situations and to access specialized care. (I get similar requests almost every week in my inbox.) This organization is called Treatment and Research Advancements National Association for Borderline Personality Disorder (TARA4BPD; https://www.tara4bpd.org/).

Another line of intervention is related to these forms of advocacy. Not everyone will read a whole book on BPD, even a short one. Families need to learn about how to manage members who have the disorder and how not to make things worse. Some of this work can be done by therapists. My city has organizations that offer support and education in groups, and they are supported by public funds and charities.

The internet also provides good information on BPD that families can use. (However, I am sorry to say that some websites are not very reputable, focusing on the most dangerous scenarios that tend to scare patients away.) McLean Hospital, linked to Harvard University, has long been a world leader in BPD treatment and research. Their website provides an accurate and readable summary called "Everything You Need to Know About Borderline Personality Disorder" (https://www.mcleanhospital.org/essential/bpd). This site also offers free webinars. It also includes some good advice for parents of a child with BPD, emphasizing how to replace critical invalidation with supportive validation and support. Another useful site with up-to-date information on BPD for patients and their families is offered by the National Institute for Mental Health (https://www.nimh.nih.gov/health/topics/borderline-personality-disorder).

Therapists should also consider meeting families to transmit some of this common-sense guidance. We do not do so routinely, because patients do not always want their families involved. But if you have the perception of only one person in a family of what is going on, and that perception is distorted by emotion dysregulation in the face of disappointments of all kinds, you will have some surprises when you meet the parents of a BPD patient. Only a minority are toxic to the point of traumatizing their children. Most are well meaning but befuddled by psychological problems. They have done all the things that parents do for their children but do not understand their special needs, in particular the need for emotional validation. They can benefit from support as well as advice about how to communicate with children who are exquisitely sensitive to even a hint of invalidation. Programs that help these families will also bring the day closer when, as often happens, there can be a reconciliation based on lower expectations on both sides.

## SUMMARY POINTS

- Psychotherapy for BPD tends to be lengthy, expensive, and not widely available.
- Briefer methods using a stepped care model have the potential to provide access to more patients.
- Families of BPD patients can benefit from support and skill training.

# 6 THE PROBLEM OF SUICIDALITY

In this chapter, I address the problem of chronic suicidality in borderline personality disorder (BPD). There is no evidence that hospitalizing patients with BPD is effective for the prevention of suicide. Instead, I propose an approach to this clinical problem that focuses more on empathy, respect, and patience in the conduct of psychotherapy.

## CHRONIC SUICIDALITY AND HOW IT DIFFERS FROM ACUTE SUICIDALITY

Patients with BPD can think about suicide for years. They often make suicide attempts, and somewhere between 5% and 10% eventually die by their own hand (Paris, 2003, 2020c, 2023b). Thus, suicidality can be a question of life or death and, when chronic, is an even more difficult problem—for those who suffer from it, for their families, and for clinicians. I know of therapists who refuse to treat such cases because they feel trapped by the threat of suicide and/or because they fear being held responsible if the patient dies.

https://doi.org/10.1037/0000440-007
*A Concise Guide to Borderline Personality Disorder*, by J. Paris

In actuality, all mental health clinicians have to deal with the possibility that some of their clients will die by suicide. A therapist who has never had a patient die by suicide is not treating seriously ill patients.

Therapists may also feel forced to do things for suicidal patients that are not helpful and that may even be counterproductive. They have been trained to follow clinical practice guidelines and were taught strategies believed to provide suicide prevention. Most of these guidelines advise that patients who threaten to commit suicide or make attempts need to be seen in emergency rooms (ERs), hospitalized, or both. But that recommendation is not evidence based. It makes sense in other major mental disorders, for which there is treatment that requires a hospital setting. Of course, BPD patients can also choose to go to a hospital on their own, usually when they feel they cannot control the emotions that lead them to consider suicide, but there are no data showing that suicide can be prevented by an admission, whether brief or long term. In the absence of such evidence, sending patients with BPD to an ER can be unhelpful.

You may find this conclusion surprising. But just spend a few hours in a crowded and overflowing ER, where patients wait hours to be evaluated and then are usually sent home. If you do, you may well reach the same conclusion.

This is not to say that hospitalization for suicidality is always a mistake. There are exceptions. The most severe mental disorders, such as melancholic depression, bipolarity, and schizophrenia, all have high rates of death by suicide, between 5% and 10% (Moitra et al., 2021). These cases may well require an admission, but not necessarily to prevent suicide. These mental disorders respond to pharmacological treatment that demand close monitoring on an inpatient unit. Patients with melancholic depression benefit from staying on wards where they can receive medication and/or electroconvulsive therapy, which work to control severe mood disorders.

BPD patients, however, do not benefit from any of these options. There is no specific pharmacological or biological treatment for the disorder. The most treatments with the strongest evidence base are better carried out over time in outpatient settings. Moreover, patients do not get effective therapy on many wards, where they may spend the day on their phones or watching television. Even if patients have an overnight stay in the ER, there is little to do but wait. When they are finally seen, they will be asked about suicidal intent, which is not a useful predictor of a fatal outcome (Franklin et al., 2017). If they give the "wrong" answer, they may be kept until they give the "right" one. I am not alone among BPD experts in avoiding admissions to a hospital or sending patients to an ER (Gunderson & Links, 2014; Linehan, 1993; Maltsberger, 1994a, 1994b).

Again, there are a few exceptions. Clinicians should consider a brief admission for a BPD patient after a life-threatening suicide attempt, to evaluate a life situation in more detail and to meet with family members. If a patient is having a brief psychotic episode, treatment with medication will be more effective in an inpatient setting.

However, suicidal ideas and attempts by themselves do not usually benefit from an admission. The point is that in BPD, mood is highly unstable, and these patients suffer from chronic suicidality. They may consider suicide on a daily basis for years. Even when not in crisis, the option of suicide remains in the back of their minds. We need to understand this clinical picture to treat it.

I would like, as I have in previous books, to quote a patient who recovered from BPD (Williams, 1998) and published her own take on what happens when chronic suicidality is routinely treated as an acute life-threatening episode:

> Do not hospitalize a person with borderline personality disorder for more than 48 hours. My self-destructive episodes—one leading right into another—came out only after my first and subsequent hospital admissions, after I learned the system was usually obligated to respond. (p. 174)

This quote offers an inside picture of suicidality in BPD. Patients may not intend to die when they describe suicidality but are instead seeking validation of their distress. If reinforced by our interventions, it can lead to a pattern of recurrent ER visits and hospitalizations. This result is all too common, but it does little for patients.

## NONSUICIDAL SELF-INJURY

Nonsuicidal self-injury (NSSI) is, by definition, not suicidal behavior. I discuss it here because it is sometimes seen that way and because people who self-harm may also threaten suicide. This pattern of behavior usually begins in adolescence. It involves wrist-cutting that is not deep enough to be dangerous. Patients usually describe feeling relief from negative emotions when they cut (Linehan, 1993). Thus, like so many other features of BPD, symptoms begin with emotion dysregulation that leads to self-harm. This behavior is adopted because it works, at least temporarily. It is for that reason that NSSI can become addictive.

NSSI was not too common until the past few decades, when its prevalence has increased. This is most likely due to *social contagion*, behaviors that spread within peer groups (Nock, 2010). Today, the internet is the vehicle for the spread of this pattern. Epidemiological studies of adolescents in the

United States have confirmed that NSSI has been on the increase and that it now has a 12-month community prevalence of 7.3%, with similar findings noted in other developed countries (Cha et al., 2018; Nock, 2010).

Adolescents can learn about NSSI online through social media, or they can be influenced by their social networks (Jarvi et al., 2013). However, long-term follow-up studies show that most adolescents with NSSI give up cutting over time and that it is most often intermittent and experimental; only a minority continue this behavior into adulthood (Moran et al., 2012). However, as our own research has shown, those who continue to self-harm have higher levels of emotion dysregulation at baseline and are at risk of developing BPD (Biskin et al., 2021).

We live in an age when ideas, both good and bad, travel at the speed of light. Adolescents with dysregulated emotions are vulnerable to self-harm because it is one way of dealing with distress. This may be an example of how the internet has been a powerful medium for social contagion. Although self-harm behaviors may initially be hidden, they offer a respite from emotion dysregulation. The mechanism behind NSSI uses physical pain as a distraction from mental pain. Unfortunately, some patients end up having permanent scars and need to wear long sleeves in warm weather. It is rare to see patients who still cut at age 30. Although NSSI can be one of the early behavioral patterns of BPD in adolescent populations, it usually remits with time (Moran et al., 2012; Nock, 2010).

In short, NSSI is a maladaptive way of dealing with emotion dysregulation. Unfortunately, relief is temporary, and the causes of distress often are not addressed.

## UNDERSTANDING CHRONIC SUICIDALITY

Suicide is the main reason why I became interested in BPD as a young clinician. It was hard for me to understand why patients would ever feel suicidal. As reviewed by Reeves et al., 2022, about 10% of the U.S. adult population report having had suicidal ideation, while 90% have not. I remember as a medical intern seeing colleagues furious with patients coming to the ER after an overdose. As they saw it, if they work hard to save lives, they perceived no need to feel sympathetic to people who want to throw their lives away. I understand this reaction, but I see suicidality as a challenge, not a reason to deny treatment.

A better way to frame suicidality is through an ability to imagine what it is like to be in severe and unremitting psychological pain. We all know what it is to like to suffer physical pain: If it is bad enough, people can feel that they would do almost anything to make it stop. Psychological pain that goes on for years can be just as hard to tolerate (Shneidman, 1996). The wish to escape, by whatever means, may then take precedence.

For most people, even after painful life experiences there are always reasons for living (Malone et al., 2000). These reasons usually derive from attachments to other people, a need to protect family members and other loved ones, and a commitment to a meaningful job or career. We are a social species, and what people most care about is each other. But when a series of relationships have failed, when a cherished job is lost, the sense of connection to the wider world can seem entirely lost.

The key to understanding chronic suicidality is a paradox. Many patients with BPD need to retain the option of suicide. When they feel they have no power over their life, they retain the choice of dying (Maltsberger, 1994a, 1994b). Clinicians should therefore be cautious about challenging this coping mechanism too soon. Patients with BPD may prefer to retain suicidal ideas until they feel in control of their life and their fate. The knowledge that they can choose to die allows them to go on living.

CASE EXAMPLE 6.1
## CHRONIC SUICIDALITY

Moira was a 35-year-old woman working as an administrative assistant for a business who was highly competent in her work. She had never attempted suicide but had seriously considered it over many years. Moira had little support from family and had been estranged from her alcoholic mother for years. She lacked close friends, and often lost them because of her angry responses to disappointment. Moira had one unsuccessful long-term relationship with a man who was addicted to cocaine, and most of her intimate connections lasted only a few months. When asked by one of her clinicians if she was willing to give up the option of suicide temporarily in order to focus on building a life worth living, she stated that doing so was out of the question.

This vignette is an example of how chronic suicidality can function as a defense against rejection and mental pain.

## WHY CLINICIANS CANNOT PREDICT OR PREVENT DEATH BY SUICIDE

Because suicide is almost always a tragedy, much has been written about how to prevent it. However, although many attempts at prediction have been suggested, experts in suicide research agree that a fatal outcome in patients is not foreseeable in any practical way (O'Connor & Pirkis, 2016). And if you cannot predict suicide, you cannot prevent it. Let us see why this is the case.

First, the term "suicidality" covers a lot of ground. It may just refer to suicidal ideation, which is fairly common. As shown in epidemiological surveys, in any given year about 3% of the population will be troubled by thoughts of suicide, and 13.5% will have had these thoughts at some point in their lifetime (Kessler, Berglund, et al., 2005). However, because not every depressed person considers suicide, the rate of suicidal ideation is lower than the community prevalence of major depression, which is about 9% in a year and at least 30% over a lifetime (Kessler, Chiu, et al., 2005). The prevalence of suicide attempts in the community is even lower: In the large-scale National Comorbidity Survey, it was 4.6% over a lifetime (Kessler, Berglund, et al., 2005). However, that rate includes a wide range of incidents, from impulsive gestures to life-threatening behaviors.

How useful is suicidality as a marker to predict the risk for a fatal outcome? The current suicide rate in the United States (as of 2021) is 14 per 100,000, that is, 0.014 (Ehlman et al., 2022). This number reflects the enormous discrepancy between thoughts (rather common), attempts (present in only a minority), and mortality (comparatively rare). These data tell us something important, which is that suicidality is too common, and death by suicide too rare to allow for useful predictions. You cannot predict a rare outcome from risk factors that are much more ubiquitous.

For example, a long-term follow-up of patients who attempted suicide in ERs found that only 3% eventually died, and 97% went on living (Hawton et al., 2003). This finding is robust in the research literature and suggests that attempted suicide is usually ambivalent and that it performs a different function.

Decades ago, Beautrais (2001) wrote a seminal article pointing out that those who attempt and those who complete suicide are different but overlapping populations. In other words, most people who attempt suicide are expressing distress but are ambivalent about dying. That is why those who attempt suicide, who are mostly women, seek treatment and often make attempts that are nonlethal. In contrast, studies of those who have completed suicide find that only a minority had sought help (McGirr et al., 2007). Those who do complete suicide are most often men, who use methods such as firearms and hanging. For this reason, most suicidal men die on the first attempt. Treatment-seeking patients usually involve overdoses of pills, the majority of which are not life threatening. These patients have been studied in follow-ups of people who attempted suicide who were seen in the ER (Hawton et al., 2003).

These observations have important implications for BPD. This is a clinical population that mostly consists of women who may repeatedly attempt suicide yet choose to go on living. We have a good chance of helping these patients, because they are looking for treatment. Moreover, the effectiveness of therapy for suicidality has been confirmed by meta-analyses (Calati & Courtet, 2016; Meerwijk et al., 2016). But getting patients to give up the idea of suicide is not suicide prevention, because most deaths occur in people who do not seek therapy. Although a history of previous attempts is a statistically significant risk factor, it is not a useful predictor of who will or will not die. The reason is that most people who make attempts do not die by suicide.

The pathway to suicide prevention with the strongest evidence base is a population approach that focuses on removing access to fatal means. There are many ways to achieve that goal (Paris, 2023b). Physicians can prescribe drugs in small amounts. Barriers on bridges can be built (the Golden Gate Bridge in San Francisco now has one). For those most at risk of a fatal outcome, the most useful intervention could be gun control. Although controlling access to guns is not currently possible in countries such as the United States, where many oppose it, this is a strategy that would have a real impact on the largely male groups who die on their first attempt and who have not necessarily received mental health treatment. The other method commonly used by men who die by suicide is hanging, but it is hard to imagine barring access to ropes.

## MANAGING SUICIDALITY IN PSYCHOTHERAPY

Research findings on the unpredictability of suicide should not be seen as discouraging. On the contrary, I see this literature as reassuring. If most patients who consider suicide choose to go on living, and if we cannot predict who will eventually chose to die, the outcome, whether life or of death, is not under our control. We need not worry excessively over the possibility of events that are bound to happen in certain cases but occur relatively rarely in a clinician's career. This knowledge can free us to concentrate on our job as therapists.

The problem is that suicidal crises are frightening. (Even after over 50 years of experience, I find these situations anxiety provoking.) Some patients with a strong need to die may come close to death, requiring medical treatment in an intensive care unit. However, multiple longitudinal follow-ups have shown that even patients who require that level of care do not necessarily die in the end (Zanarini, 2019). In fact, suicides often occur within a month or a few months after discharge from the hospital (Chung et al., 2017; Haglund et al., 2019). Yet although about 10% of patients admitted to hospital will end their lives by suicide at some later point, 70% will not make any further attempts (Owens et al., 2002).

All this evidence explains why I am generally opposed to hospitalization for suicidality in BPD. Most experts on the disorder agree with me (Choi-Kain & Gunderson, 2019; Livesley, 2017). Linehan (1993) is also skeptical about the value of admission to a hospital but suggested that an overnight hold can be face-saving. About 20 years ago, at a meeting of the American Psychiatric Association, I heard Dr. Linehan make an ironic remark that it might be better for BPD patients if ERs were nasty places where nobody would want to go. And some of my colleagues from the United States think that the limited insurance coverage for hospitalization in that country has been a boon for BPD patients, who can usually be safely sent home after a brief hold in the ER or a ward.

Again, I allow for some exceptions. When suicidal episodes have come close to fatality, a hospitalization provides a useful breather during which to review the treatment plan. However, this does not prove that hospitalization can prevent suicide. Fortunately, most suicide attempts in BPD patients consist of nonlethal overdoses. Moreover, keep in mind that cutting and related forms of self-harm are rarely suicidal in intent (Brown et al., 2002). A few patients cut themselves deeply enough to need stitches, or even open up an artery, but these scenarios are uncommon. What clinicians face in practice in managing suicidality is not so much the threat of death but a persistent picture of turmoil associated with emotion dysregulation.

Managing suicidality is hard work, but that is not a reason to refuse access to therapy. In my own case, I feel a responsibility to pay back a debt to society, which invested in my training to be a physician and a psychiatrist. Many of my nonmedical colleagues are understandably spooked by suicidality, in part because they have not had training in the management of death and dying. As a researcher on BPD, I consider it my duty to take on patients in my practice who are at greatest risk. I no longer treat patients who do not have a severe personality disorder.

Keep in mind that the wish to die in BPD patients is typically ambivalent. Most patients will either contact someone else in their social network to bring them to the hospital or anticipate that someone will find them in time. But some attempts are a kind of Russian roulette, in which whether a patient can or cannot be saved becomes a matter of chance. It is not clear that we can prevent suicide in such cases.

What I propose is that although the treatment of chronically suicidal patients begins with an acceptance by both parties that suicide remains an option, therapy offers an opportunity to find reasons for living. The patient needs only to agree that doing so is worth a try, even if they retain the option of suicide. (It may also be useful to have a similar conversation with family members if patients agree to them being involved.) And people who come for help do not necessarily want to remain suicidal. Over the years, I have treated hundreds of patients with BPD, but only four of them died by suicide while in therapy. (A few others died years later, when no longer in treatment.) As I discussed in Chapter 2, a minority of patients who do not improve with treatment are more at risk.

Therapy for suicidality need not be much different from the treatment principles described in Chapter 5, but patients can be told that before committing to death, it is worth giving life a chance. This means learning better skills in handling emotions and relationships. In other words, we respect our patients' autonomy by not excluding suicide as an option but encourage them to postpone any decision until therapy is well underway.

A new wrinkle for therapists who work with this population is the availability of assisted suicide in the medical system (Steck et al., 2013). Until recently, that option was available only to patients with incurable and fatal diseases that have death as a predictable outcome. However, a few European countries, and some American states, have opened up assisted suicide to psychiatric patients who suffer in a different way. As we have seen, that kind of distress can be severe, and it is termed *psychache* (Shneidman, 1996). But it is wrong to consider psychological pain incurable.

As I write, Canada has been considering whether to expand its policy of "medical aid in dying" to psychiatric patients who have not recovered from an illness (Nicolini et al., 2020). I consider this proposal to be a serious error. One cannot say with any degree of certainty that chronically suicidal patients will never recover, or that any of the conditions we treat are—in the wording of the proposed law, "irremediable." In most cases, even among the most severely ill patients, the trajectory of BPD moves toward recovery (Zanarini, 2019). Moreover, medical aid in dying could be used as a substitute for care when resources are limited (Appelbaum, 2024).

Most psychiatrists will refuse to be involved in such a procedure: In the countries where medically assisted dying has been legalized (e.g., the Netherlands, Belgium, Switzerland), only a few clinicians have been willing to do this kind of work. However, after most Canadian psychiatrists expressed their opposition, and provincial health ministries indicated doubt about whether such a project could work, it has been postponed (at least for now; Shannon et al., 2023).

A final issue concerns the fear among clinicians of being sued by family members for malpractice if a patient dies by suicide. This is a threat that is frightening to all who treat these patients. However, although this scenario is one of the leading causes of lawsuits against mental health professionals, it is not that common, and the vast majority of such claims are rejected by the courts (Gutheil, 1992). Gutheil (2004) usefully recommended ways to limit liability: that families be contacted early in therapy if the risk is high, that careful records be kept, and that consultations be requested and their results faithfully recorded. Some hospitals, in particular in the United States, where litigation is higher than in other countries, are concerned about their legal liability, yet this view of the problem could be counterproductive if active therapy is derailed by multiple admissions. In summary, although there are times when admission to a hospital is unavoidable, we need to keep the long-term consequences of doing so in mind.

CASE EXAMPLE 6.2
## SUICIDAL IDEATION ONLY

Norma was a law student with a psychiatric history that went back to her early adolescent years. Even though she had several brief hospital admissions, her problems did not affect her studies. Norma had seen several experienced therapists without much benefit, and her dramatic but chronic suicidality usually led to some degree of therapist burnout. She was not respectful of boundaries, and on one occasion, when her therapist was recovering in the hospital after surgery, she visited him there to start a dialogue about how difficult she found being without him. On other occasions, she would repeatedly call therapists with blood-curdling suicidal threats. Norma was offered many medications, but although she took them she would hear critical voices in her head. Despite these difficulties, Norma matured with time and finished her education. As was shown by a long-term follow-up interview at age 40, she had success working in a law firm and even got married and had children.

CASE EXAMPLE 6.3
## DANGEROUS SUICIDE ATTEMPTS

Olivia was a 35-year-old woman working at a call center. Her long psychiatric history included near-fatal suicide attempts that had led to multiple hospitalizations as well as self-harm marked by deep and dangerous cutting. On one occasion, while in our program, she left group therapy to overdose on pills in a nearby bathroom. Oliva had severe emotion dysregulation and on a few occasions had to be removed by the police from shops where she had gone into uncontrollable rages. Nonetheless, she kept some friends, and she had an on-and-off boyfriend. At a 10-year follow-up, Olivia was no longer suicidal and was working regularly.

CASE EXAMPLE 6.4

## SUICIDALITY WITH MICROPSYCHOSIS

Paula was a 16-year-old girl who came to see me after her best friend died after jumping off a bridge. Paula had long considered doing the same thing, and the friend had suggested they jump together. Paula's family was dysfunctional, with an alcoholic father who sexually abused her and a mother who was unable to look after her, leading her to seek refuge by living in the house of her older, married sister. Paula also had a vivid fantasy life, hearing voices and imagining herself as living on another planet. These micropsychotic features, as well as her chronic suicidality, had led to a brief hospital admission. However, at a 20-year follow-up Paula reported that she had largely recovered. She was now married with children, held a steady job, and advocated for troubled children by sitting on a school board.

CASE EXAMPLE 6.5

## FATALITY

Roberta was a 40-year-old woman working in a bank. She had suffered from suicidal ideas since childhood and had a history of polysubstance abuse during her adolescence and youth. Nonetheless, Roberta was university educated, with a successful career. However, she was unable to accept rejection from her boyfriend of 5 years, who left her because of her emotionality. However, none of the multiple therapists she saw over the next few years, including one who was part of a dialectical behavior therapy program, was able to help her. Roberta stated she could not find reasons for living, especially without love. She was then admitted to a hospital and given a course of ketamine infusions to manage what the psychiatrists there had considered to be treatment-resistant depression, but this treatment was also not helpful. She then entered our program but died of an overdose after attending 1 month of group and individual therapy. The therapist met with her parents, who were understandably sad and angry about this outcome but who reported that, in spite of their best intentions, they had never been able to get through to her.

CASE EXAMPLE 6.6
## RECOVERY AFTER A NEAR-FATAL ATTEMPT

Theresa was a 29-year-old woman working in a computer company who was now in her second marriage. Her relationships had always been stormy, and she had long suffered from mood swings. Her first marriage had ended when her husband said he could no longer deal with her needs, and the second was already turning out much the same. But Theresa always seemed to need a man in her life. After a bad quarrel with her husband, she took a very large overdose. Her husband found her unconscious, and she was treated in an intensive care unit for several days, followed by an admission to a psychiatric unit. Eventually, after being treated for 1 year in our program, Theresa reinvested in her career goals and married again, this time to an older man for whom she had been working. At a 10-year follow-up she was already a widow but now deeply involved in the care of a nephew who had a chronic genetic illness. She was no longer thinking of suicide.

Chronic suicidality is one of the greatest challenges mental health professionals face; however, the outcome is not predictable, and most patients never die by their own hand. This form of suicidality can best be understood as an attempt to control one's fate in a world that is seen as both unsupportive and dangerous.

## SUMMARY POINTS

- Chronic suicidality is different from the more acute forms seen in depression.
- There is no evidence that suicide can be prevented in BPD patients. Hospitalization has not been shown to prevent fatal outcomes.
- Suicidal ideas can be considered as a defense that a patient will give up only when reasons for living become stronger than reasons for dying.

# 7 SUMMARY AND FUTURE DIRECTIONS

There has been great progress over several decades in understanding and treating borderline personality disorder (BPD). In this chapter, I emphasize that this increased optimism needs to be translated into greater levels of accessibility to evidence-based treatment.

## SUMMARY OF THE MAIN POINTS OF THIS BOOK

- BPD is a major public health problem. The disorder is often seen in practice and is characterized by emotion dysregulation, impulsivity, and problematic relationships.

- BPD could be labeled with a different name, but the problems associated with this disorder will not go away if were. It is possible that the diagnosis of BPD will be changed once its etiology is thoroughly understood, but most clinicians are not yet convinced that scoring patients on trait profiles can provide a better guideline to treatment than the current system.

https://doi.org/10.1037/0000440-008
*A Concise Guide to Borderline Personality Disorder*, by J. Paris

- BPD is a disorder of adolescence that usually gets better with time. For most patients, BPD can be readily diagnosed at an early age, after which a period of turmoil over the next few years typically follows. Yet although patients continue to have difficulties early in life, very few meet the criteria for this diagnosis after early middle age. The disorder can sometimes be chronic, but most patients have a good prognosis and can be expected to recover.

- Like other mental disorders, BPD is the proverbial elephant that can be described in different ways by different observers, each of which focuses on a single aspect of the problem. Most clinicians prefer simplicity to complexity and find it harder to think in terms of interactions and easier to assume single pathways to disorder. However, BPD is a syndrome that has no single cause. It can be understood only in the context of a biopsychosocial model.

- It would be helpful if neuroscience researchers could discover specific changes in brain function involved in the development of BPD, but just about every research tool has been applied to this search without yielding anything that comes close to a definitive answer. Perhaps future technology can eventually do better, but that is a task for a century, not for a decade.

- BPD is not mainly caused by childhood trauma, although it tends to be worsened by child abuse. Emotional neglect, a history that can be found in almost all patients, is the most important early adversity. A biosocial model of the disorder emphasizes interactions between heritable traits of emotion dysregulation and the invalidation of these emotions by significant others. This model extends this view, taking into account social forces that make BPD symptoms more prevalent.

- We now know that BPD can, in most cases, be treated successfully with psychotherapy. Although dialectical behavior therapy has the most research behind it, a set of alternatives that can accomplish much the same thing is available. This suggests a need for a single integrative model to replace acronym-based methods.

- BPD does not respond well to any of the medications that are used for patients with other mental health conditions. With the exception of insomnia, most patients can be managed without psychopharmacology. This conclusion could change in the future, but at present BPD patients are widely overmedicated with drugs designed for other purposes.

- BPD patients can think about suicide for years, often make attempts, and frequently present to hospital emergency rooms with suicidality. Although somewhere between 5% and 10% eventually take their own life, the good news is that at least 90% decide to go on living (Paris, 2003; Zanarini, 2019). Suicide is always a risk in BPD, but attempts to prevent it can sometimes be counterproductive. Therapists need to understand that suicidality serves a psychological function for patients, as an escape from mental pain.

- Because of the severity of this disorder and the demand on clinical services, BPD remains a primary focus of research on personality disorders. As a soldier in a large army of investigators, I can confirm we have learned a great deal in the past 50 years, but this has entailed gradual progress rather than a dramatic breakthrough. Treating BPD patients is not easy, but because most patients respond to treatment the work is rewarding. Recovery largely depends on finding reasons for living.

## FUTURE DIRECTIONS

We are just at the beginning of a long road that will eventually lead to a better understanding of BPD. The biopsychosocial theory developed in this book should be considered a first step. Its main advantage is that it avoids vast oversimplifications, such as "BPD is a form of posttraumatic stress disorder arising from childhood trauma" or "BPD is a mood disorder arising from genetically determined brain abnormalities." Such narrow points of view show us how hard it is for clinicians (and researchers) to address complex problems with interactive models. Yes, BPD is often associated with childhood trauma, but only a minority of patients have that history (Porter et al., 2020), and yes, BPD is partly heritable and is associated with variations in brain circuitry. But these features do not predict, by themselves, the development of the disorder. BPD is a complex illness with symptoms in all domains of psychopathology. There is no single pathway to BPD; instead, there is a range of risk factors that are additive and interactive.

Those of us who study severe mental disorders know that our present lack of detailed knowledge is by no means unique. After decades of extensive research, we still have little idea why people develop schizophrenia or bipolar disorders. When it comes to diseases of the brain, we are looking at defects in a neural system that may be the most complex in the known universe, with 86 billion neurons linked by many trillions of synapses. It will take many decades before we have theories that explain psychopathology in the human brain. We have many blank spaces that require better theories and much more data. A focus on biological risks alone, psychological risks alone, or social risks alone will not be sufficient. This book aims to debunk such simplistic theories.

The prognosis for BPD treatment is now reasonably optimistic. The main problem is the failure to recognize that patients with chronic anxiety and/or depression often have personality disorders. Today, word has gotten around that patients usually recover and that most respond to well-planned psychotherapy, but I still see many cases in which multiple medications or genetic therapies have been tried for long periods and failed. The problem here lies with clinicians and their preconceptions. As the saying goes, if you have a hammer, everything looks like a nail. But BPD requires more sophisticated interventions than standard therapies and medications. It is one of a set of conditions that, like addictions and eating disorders, may require management by a specialized team. Although mental health services these days are stretched, much time can be wasted offering the wrong treatment to people with personality disorders. We also know that once a diagnosis is made, there are now effective options at our disposal.

I have emphasized in this book that even if we have good treatments for BPD, they require large investments in human resources, that is, courses of therapy that are effective as well as accessible and affordable. This is a problem for the mental health system as a whole, not just for BPD. Many treatments are not adequately covered by health insurance, and even those that are may not have a strong evidence base. Although we have seen real progress, the persistent stigma of mental illness still stands in our way.

We live in a time when cases of BPD, long considered untreatable, can usually be managed successfully. Clinicians should not be afraid to take on these challenging but fascinating patients.

# References

Amad, A., Ramoz, N., Thomas, P., Jardri, R., & Gorwood, P. (2014). Genetics of borderline personality disorder: Systematic review and proposal of an integrative model. *Neuroscience and Biobehavioral Reviews, 40*, 6–19. https://doi.org/10.1016/j.neubiorev.2014.01.003

American Psychiatric Association. (1952). *Diagnostic and statistical manual of mental disorders.*

American Psychiatric Association. (1968). *Diagnostic and statistical manual of mental disorders* (2nd ed.).

American Psychiatric Association. (1980). *Diagnostic and statistical manual of mental disorders* (3rd ed.).

American Psychiatric Association. (1994). *Diagnostic and statistical manual of mental disorders* (4th ed.).

American Psychiatric Association. (2013). *Diagnostic and statistical manual of mental disorders* (5th ed.). https://doi.org/10.1176/appi.books.9780890425596

American Psychiatric Association. (2022). *Diagnostic and statistical manual of mental disorders* (5th ed., text rev.). https://doi.org/10.1176/appi.books.9780890425787

Appelbaum, P. S. (2024). Physician-assisted death for psychiatric disorders: Ongoing reasons for concern. *World Psychiatry, 23*(1), 56–57. https://doi.org/10.1002/wps.21153

Asarnow, J. R., Berk, M. S., Bedics, J., Adrian, M., Gallop, R., Cohen, J., Korslund, K., Hughes, J., Avina, C., Linehan, M. M., & McCauley, E. (2021). Dialectical behavior therapy for suicidal self-harming youth: Emotion regulation, mechanisms, and mediators. *Journal of the American Academy of Child & Adolescent Psychiatry, 60*(9), 1105–1115.e4. https://doi.org/10.1016/j.jaac.2021.01.016

Assary, E., Vincent, J. P., Keers, R., & Pluess, M. (2018). Gene–environment interaction and psychiatric disorders: Review and future directions. *Seminars in Cell & Developmental Biology, 77*, 133–143. https://doi.org/10.1016/j.semcdb.2017.10.016

Barkham, M., Lutz, W., & Castonguay, L. G. (Eds.). (2021). *Bergin and Garfield's handbook of psychotherapy and behavior change* (50th Anniv. ed.). Wiley.

Barkley, R. A. (2019). Neuropsychological testing is not useful in the diagnosis of ADHD: Stop it (or prove it)! *The ADHD Report, 27*(2), 1–8. https://doi.org/10.1521/adhd.2019.27.2.1

Barkley, R. A., Murphy, K. R., & Fischer, M. (2010). *ADHD in adults: What the science says*. Guilford Press.

Barnicot, K., & Crawford, M. (2019). Dialectical behaviour therapy v. mentalisation-based therapy for borderline personality disorder. *Psychological Medicine, 49*(12), 2060–2068. https://doi.org/10.1017/S0033291718002878

Barrigón, M. L., Diaz, F. J., Gurpegui, M., Ferrin, M., Salcedo, M. D., Moreno-Granados, J., Cervilla, J. A., & Ruiz-Veguilla, M. (2015). Childhood trauma as a risk factor for psychosis: A sib-pair study. *Journal of Psychiatric Research, 70*, 130–136. https://doi.org/10.1016/j.jpsychires.2015.08.017

Barsaglini, A., Sartori, G., Benetti, S., Pettersson-Yeo, W., & Mechelli, A. (2014). The effects of psychotherapy on brain function: A systematic and critical review. *Progress in Neurobiology, 114*, 1–14. https://doi.org/10.1016/j.pneurobio.2013.10.006

Bateman, A., Constantinou, M. P., Fonagy, P., & Holzer, S. (2021). Eight-year prospective follow-up of mentalization-based treatment versus structured clinical management for people with borderline personality disorder. *Personality Disorders: Theory, Research, and Treatment, 12*(4), 291–299. https://doi.org/10.1037/per0000422

Bateman, A., & Fonagy, P. (1999). Effectiveness of partial hospitalization in the treatment of borderline personality disorder: A randomized controlled trial. *The American Journal of Psychiatry, 156*(10), 1563–1569. https://doi.org/10.1176/ajp.156.10.1563

Bateman, A., & Fonagy, P. (2004). *Psychotherapy for borderline personality disorder: Mentalization based treatment*. Oxford University Press. https://doi.org/10.1093/med:psych/9780198527664.001.0001

Bateman, A., & Fonagy, P. (2006). *Mentalization based treatment: A practical guide*. Wiley.

Bateman, A., & Fonagy, P. (2008). 8-year follow-up of patients treated for borderline personality disorder: Mentalization-based treatment versus treatment as usual. *The American Journal of Psychiatry, 165*(5), 631–638. https://doi.org/10.1176/appi.ajp.2007.07040636

Bateman, A., & Fonagy, P. (2009). Randomized controlled trial of outpatient mentalization-based treatment versus structured clinical management for borderline personality disorder. *The American Journal of Psychiatry, 166*(12), 1355–1364. https://doi.org/10.1176/appi.ajp.2009.09040539

Beauchaine, T. P., & Cicchetti, D. (2019). Emotion dysregulation and emerging psychopathology: A transdiagnostic, transdisciplinary perspective. *Development and Psychopathology, 31*(3), 799–804. https://doi.org/10.1017/S0954579419000671

Beautrais, A. L. (2001). Suicides and serious suicide attempts: Two populations or one? *Psychological Medicine, 31*(5), 837–845. https://doi.org/10.1017/S0033291701003889

Becker, L. G., Asadi, S., Zimmerman, M., Morgan, T. A., & Rodriguez-Seijas, C. (2023). Is there a bias in the diagnosis of borderline personality disorder among racially minoritized patients? *Personality Disorders: Theory, Research, and Treatment, 14*(3), 339–346. https://doi.org/10.1037/per0000579

Bedics, J. (Ed.). (2020). *The handbook of dialectical behavior therapy: Theory, research and evaluation*. Academic Press.

Belsky, J., & Pluess, M. (2009). The nature (and nurture?) of plasticity in early human development. *Perspectives on Psychological Science, 4*(4), 345–351. https://doi.org/10.1111/j.1745-6924.2009.01136.x

Benedetti, F. (2020). *Placebo effects* (3rd ed.). Oxford University Press. https://doi.org/10.1093/oso/9780198843177.001.0001

Bhugra, D., Moussaoui, D., & Craig, T. J. (Eds.). (2022). *Oxford textbook of social psychiatry*. Oxford University Press. https://doi.org/10.1093/med/9780198861478.001.0001

Binks, C. A., Fenton, M., McCarthy, L., Lee, T., Adams, C. E., & Duggan, C. (2006). Pharmacological interventions for people with borderline personality disorder. *Cochrane Database of Systematic Reviews*. https://doi.org/10.1002/14651858.CD005653

Biskin, R. S., Paris, J., Renaud, J., Raz, A., & Zelkowitz, P. (2011). Outcomes in women diagnosed with borderline personality disorder in adolescence. *Journal of the Canadian Academy of Child and Adolescent Psychiatry, 20*(3), 168–174.

Biskin, R. S., Paris, J., Zelkowitz, P., Mills, D., Laporte, L., & Heath, N. (2021). Nonsuicidal self-injury in early adolescence as a predictor of borderline personality disorder features in early adulthood. *Journal of Personality Disorders, 35*(5), 764–775. https://doi.org/10.1521/pedi_2020_34_500

Black, D. W., Zanarini, M. C., Romine, A., Shaw, M., Allen, J., & Schulz, S. C. (2014). Comparison of low and moderate dosages of extended-release quetiapine in borderline personality disorder: A randomized, double-blind, placebo-controlled trial. *The American Journal of Psychiatry, 171*(11), 1174–1182. https://doi.org/10.1176/appi.ajp.2014.13101348

Blum, N., St. John, D., Pfohl, B., Stuart, S., McCormick, B., Allen, J., Arndt, S., & Black, D. W. (2008). Systems Training for Emotional Predictability and Problem Solving (STEPPS) for outpatients with borderline personality disorder: A randomized controlled trial and 1-year follow-up. *The American Journal of Psychiatry, 165*(4), 468–478. https://doi.org/10.1176/appi.ajp.2007.07071079

Bornovalova, M. A., Hicks, B. M., Iacono, W. G., & McGue, M. (2009). Stability, change, and heritability of borderline personality disorder traits from adolescence to adulthood: A longitudinal twin study. *Development and Psychopathology, 21*(4), 1335–1353. https://doi.org/10.1017/S0954579409990186

Bornovalova, M., Huibregste, B. M., & Hicks, B. M. (2013). Tests of a direct effect of childhood abuse on adult borderline personality disorder traits: A longitudinal discordant twin design. *Journal of Abnormal Psychology, 122*(1), 180–194. https://doi.org/10.1037/a0028328

Bos, E. H., Van Wel, E. B., Appelo, M. T., & Verbraak, M. J. (2011). Effectiveness of Systems Training for Emotional Predictability and Problem Solving (STEPPS) for borderline personality problems in a "real-world" sample: Moderation by diagnosis or severity? *Psychotherapy and Psychosomatics, 80*(3), 173–181. https://doi.org/10.1159/000321793

Boyce, W. T. (2019). *The orchid and the dandelion: Why some children struggle and how all can thrive.* Penguin Random House.

Brettschneider, C., Riedel-Heller, S., & König, H. H. (2014). A systematic review of economic evaluations of treatments for borderline personality disorder. *PLoS One, 9*(9), e107748. https://doi.org/10.1371/journal.pone.0107748

Brown, M. Z., Comtois, K. A., & Linehan, M. M. (2002). Reasons for suicide attempts and nonsuicidal self-injury in women with borderline personality disorder. *Journal of Abnormal Psychology, 111*(1), 198–202. https://doi.org/10.1037/0021-843X.111.1.198

Brüne, M. (2001). Social cognition and psychopathology in an evolutionary perspective: Current status and proposals for research. *Psychopathology, 34*(2), 85–94. https://doi.org/10.1159/000049286

Brüne, M. (2016). Borderline personality disorder: Why "fast and furious"? *Evolution, Medicine, & Public Health, 2016*(1), 52–66. https://doi.org/10.1093/emph/eow002

Bryce, I., Pye, D., Beccaria, G., McIlveen, P., & Du Preez, J. (2023). A systematic literature review of the career choice of helping professionals who have experienced cumulative harm as a result of adverse childhood experiences. *Trauma, Violence, & Abuse, 24*(1), 72–85. https://doi.org/10.1177/15248380211016016

Bulbena-Cabre, A., Bassir Nia, A., & Perez-Rodriguez, M. M. (2018). Current knowledge on gene–environment interactions in personality disorders: An update. *Current Psychiatry Reports, 20*(9), 74–79. https://doi.org/10.1007/s11920-018-0934-7

Calati, R., & Courtet, P. (2016). Is psychotherapy effective for reducing suicide attempt and non-suicidal self-injury rates? Meta-analysis and meta-regression of literature data. *Journal of Psychiatric Research, 79*, 8–20. https://doi.org/10.1016/j.jpsychires.2016.04.003

Carlyle, D., Green, R., Inder, M., Porter, R., Crowe, M., Mulder, R., & Frampton, C. (2020). A randomized-controlled trial of mentalization-based treatment compared with structured case management for borderline personality disorder in a mainstream public health service. *Frontiers in Psychiatry, 11*, 561916. https://doi.org/10.3389/fpsyt.2020.561916

Castonguay, L. G., Eubanks, C. F., Goldfried, M. R., Muran, J. C., & Lutz, W. (2015). Research on psychotherapy integration: Building on the past, looking to the future. *Psychotherapy Research, 25*(3), 365–382. https://doi.org/10.1080/10503307.2015.1014010

Cavelti, M., Thompson, K., Chanen, A. M., & Kaess, M. (2021). Psychotic symptoms in borderline personality disorder: Developmental aspects. *Current Opinion in Psychology, 37*, 26–31. https://doi.org/10.1016/j.copsyc.2020.07.003

Cha, C. B., Franz, P. J., Guzmán, E. M., Glenn, C. R., Kleiman, E. M., & Nock, M. K. (2018). Suicide among youth—Epidemiology, (potential) etiology, and treatment. *The Journal of Child Psychology and Psychiatry, 59*(4), 460–482. https://doi.org/10.1111/jcpp.12831

Chanen, A. M. (2015). Borderline personality disorder in young people: Are we there yet? *Journal of Clinical Psychology, 71*(8), 778–791. https://doi.org/10.1002/jclp.22205

Chanen, A. M., & McCutcheon, L. (2013). Prevention and early intervention for borderline personality disorder: Current status and recent evidence. *The British Journal of Psychiatry, 202*(S54), S24–S29. https://doi.org/10.1192/bjp.bp.112.119180

Chanen, A. M., Nicol, K., Betts, J. K., & Thompson, K. N. (2020). Diagnosis and treatment of borderline personality disorder in young people. *Current Psychiatry Reports, 22*(5), Article 25. https://doi.org/10.1007/s11920-020-01144-5

Chapman, A. L. (2019). Borderline personality disorder and emotion dysregulation. *Development and Psychopathology, 31*(3), 1143–1156. https://doi.org/10.1017/S0954579419000658

Choi-Kain, L. W., Albert, E. B., & Gunderson, J. G. (2016). Evidence-based treatments for borderline personality disorder: Implementation, integration, and stepped care. *Harvard Review of Psychiatry, 24*(5), 342–356. https://doi.org/10.1097/HRP.0000000000000113

Choi-Kain, L. W., Finch, E. F., Masland, S. R., Jenkins, J. A., & Unruh, B. T. (2017). What works in the treatment of borderline personality disorder. *Current Behavioral Neuroscience Reports, 4*(1), 21–30. https://doi.org/10.1007/s40473-017-0103-z

Choi-Kain, L. W., & Gunderson, J. G. (Eds.). (2019). *Applications of good psychiatric management for borderline personality disorder: A practical guide.* American Psychiatric Publishing.

Choi-Kain, L. W., & Sharp, C. (2012). *Handbook of good psychiatric management for adolescents with borderline personality disorder.* American Psychiatric Publishing.

Choudhary, S., & Gupta, R. (2020). Culture and borderline personality disorder in India. *Frontiers in Psychology, 11*, Article 714. https://doi.org/10.3389/fpsyg.2020.00714

Chung, D. T., Ryan, C. J., Hadzi-Pavlovic, D., Singh, S. P., Stanton, C., & Large, M. M. (2017). Suicide rates after discharge from psychiatric facilities: A systematic review and meta-analysis. *JAMA Psychiatry, 74*(7), 694–702. https://doi.org/10.1001/jamapsychiatry.2017.1044

Cicchetti, D., & Rogosch, F. A. (2002). A developmental psychopathology perspective on adolescence. *Journal of Consulting and Clinical Psychology, 70*(1), 6–20. https://doi.org/10.1037/0022-006X.70.1.6

Cludius, B., Mennin, D., & Ehring, T. (2020). Emotion regulation as a transdiagnostic process. *Emotion, 20*(1), 37–42. https://doi.org/10.1037/emo0000646

Cohen, P., & Cohen, J. (1984). The clinician's illusion. *Archives of General Psychiatry, 41*(12), 1178–1182. https://doi.org/10.1001/archpsyc.1984.01790230064010

Coid, J., Yang, M., Tyrer, P., Roberts, A., & Ullrich, S. (2006). Prevalence and correlates of personality disorder in Great Britain. *The British Journal of Psychiatry, 188*(5), 423–431. https://doi.org/10.1192/bjp.188.5.423

Compton, W. M., Helzer, J. E., Hwu, H.-g., Yeh, E.-k., McEvoy, L., Tipp, J. E., & Spitznagel, E. L. (1991). New methods in cross-cultural psychiatry: Psychiatric illness in Taiwan and the United States. *The American Journal of Psychiatry, 148*(12), 1697–1704. https://doi.org/10.1176/ajp.148.12.1697

Crawford, M. J., Sanatinia, R., Barrett, B., Cunningham, G., Dale, O., Ganguli, P., Lawrence-Smith, G., Leeson, V., Lemonsky, F., Lykomitrou, G., Montgomery, A. A., Morriss, R., Munjiza, J., Paton, C., Skorodzien, I., Singh, V., Tan, W., Tyrer, P., & Reilly, J. G. (2018). The clinical effectiveness and cost-effectiveness of lamotrigine in borderline personality disorder: A randomized placebo-controlled trial. *The American Journal of Psychiatry, 175*(8), 756–764. https://doi.org/10.1176/appi.ajp.2018.17091006

Cristea, I. A., Gentili, C., Cotet, C. D., Palomba, D., Barbui, C., & Cuijpers, P. (2017). Efficacy of psychotherapies for borderline personality disorder: A systematic review and meta-analysis. *JAMA Psychiatry, 74*(4), 319–328. https://doi.org/10.1001/jamapsychiatry.2016.4287

Crotty, K., Viswanathan, M., Kennedy, S., Edlund, M. J., Ali, R., Siddiqui, M., Wines, R., Ratajczak, P., & Gartlehner, G. (2024). Psychotherapies for the treatment of borderline personality disorder: A systematic review. *Journal of Consulting and Clinical Psychology, 92*(5), 275–295. https://doi.org/10.1037/ccp0000833

Crowell, S. E., Beauchaine, T. P., & Linehan, M. M. (2009). A biosocial developmental model of borderline personality: Elaborating and extending Linehan's theory. *Psychological Bulletin, 135*(3), 495–510. https://doi.org/10.1037/a0015616

Cuthbert, B. N., & Insel, T. R. (2013). Toward the future of psychiatric diagnosis: The seven pillars of RDoC. *BMC Medicine, 11*(1), Article 126. https://doi.org/10.1186/1741-7015-11-126

Davidson, K., Norrie, J., Tyrer, P., Gumley, A., Tata, P., Murray, H., & Palmer, S. (2006). The effectiveness of cognitive behavior therapy for borderline personality disorder: Results from the Borderline Personality Disorder Study of Cognitive Therapy (BOSCOT) trial. *Journal of Personality Disorders, 20*(5), 450–465. https://doi.org/10.1521/pedi.2006.20.5.450

Del Casale, A., Bonanni, L., Bargagna, P., Novelli, F., Fiaschè, F., Paolini, M., Forcina, F., Anibaldi, G., Cortese, F. N., Iannuccelli, A., Adriani, B., Brugnoli, R., Girardi, P., Paris, J., & Pompili, M. (2021). Current clinical psychopharmacology in borderline personality disorder. *Current Neuropharmacology, 19*(10), 1760–1779. https://doi.org/10.2174/1570159X19666210610092958

Dixon-Gordon, K. L., Haliczer, L. A., & Conkey, L. C. (2020). Emotion dysregulation and borderline personality disorder. In T. P. Beauchaine & S. E. Crowell (Eds.), *The Oxford handbook of emotion dysregulation* (pp. 361–376). Oxford University Press.

Doering, S., Hörz, S., Rentrop, M., Fischer-Kern, M., Schuster, P., Benecke, C., Buchheim, A., Martius, P., & Buchheim, P. (2010). Transference-focused psychotherapy v. treatment by community psychotherapists for borderline personality disorder: Randomised controlled trial. *The British Journal of Psychiatry, 196*(5), 389–395. https://doi.org/10.1192/bjp.bp.109.070177

Domes, G., Schulze, L., & Herpertz, S. C. (2009). Emotion recognition in borderline personality disorder—A review of the literature. *Journal of Personality Disorders, 23*(1), 6–19. https://doi.org/10.1521/pedi.2009.23.1.6

Ehlman, D. C., Yard, E., Stone, D. M., Jones, C. M., & Mack, K. A. (2022). Changes in suicide rates—United States, 2019 and 2020. *Morbidity and Mortality Weekly Report, 71*(8), 306–312. https://doi.org/10.15585/mmwr.mm7108a5

Ekiz, E., van Alphen, S. P. J., Ouwens, M. A., Van de Paar, J., & Videler, A. C. (2023). Systems training for emotional predictability and problem solving for borderline personality disorder: A systematic review. *Personality and Mental Health, 17*(1), 20–39. https://doi.org/10.1002/pmh.1558

Ellison, W. D., Rosenstein, L. K., Morgan, T. A., & Zimmerman, M. (2018). Community and clinical epidemiology of borderline personality disorder. *Psychiatric Clinics of North America, 41*(4), 561–573. https://doi.org/10.1016/j.psc.2018.07.008

Engel, G. L. (1977, April 8). The need for a new medical model: A challenge for biomedicine. *Science, 196*(4286), 129–136. https://doi.org/10.1126/science.847460

Engel, G. L. (1980). The clinical application of the biopsychosocial model. *The American Journal of Psychiatry, 137*(5), 535–544. https://doi.org/10.1176/ajp.137.5.535

Fergusson, D. M., McLeod, G. F., & Horwood, L. J. (2013). Childhood sexual abuse and adult developmental outcomes: Findings from a 30-year longitudinal study in New Zealand. *Child Abuse & Neglect, 37*(9), 664–674. https://doi.org/10.1016/j.chiabu.2013.03.013

Fergusson, D. M., & Mullen, P. E. (1999). *Childhood sexual abuse* (Vol. 4). Sage.

Finch, E. F., Iliakis, E. A., Masland, S. R., & Choi-Kain, L. W. (2019). A meta-analysis of treatment as usual for borderline personality disorder. *Personality Disorders, 10*(6), 491–499. https://doi.org/10.1037/per0000353

Fok, M. L.-Y., Stewart, R., Hayes, R. D., & Moran, P. (2014). Predictors of natural and unnatural mortality among patients with personality disorder: Evidence from a large UK case register. *PLoS One, 9*(7), e100979. https://doi.org/10.1371/journal.pone.0100979

Ford, J. D., & Courtois, C. A. (2021). Complex PTSD and borderline personality disorder. *Borderline Personality Disorder and Emotion Dysregulation, 8*(1), 16–21. https://doi.org/10.1186/s40479-021-00155-9

Frances, A. (2013). *Saving normal*. HarperCollins.

Franklin, J. C., Ribeiro, J. D., Fox, K. R., Bentley, K. H., Kleiman, E. M., Huang, X., Musacchio, K. M., Jaroszewski, A. C., Chang, B. P., & Nock, M. K. (2017). Risk factors for suicidal thoughts and behaviors: A meta-analysis of 50 years of research. *Psychological Bulletin, 143*(2), 187–232. https://doi.org/10.1037/bul0000084

Fuller, J. L., & Simmel, E. C. (2023). *Perspectives in behavior genetics*. Routledge.

Gascon, A., Gamache, D., St-Laurent, D., & Stipanicic, A. (2022). Do we over-diagnose ADHD in North America? A critical review and clinical recommendations. *Journal of Clinical Psychology, 78*(12), 2363–2380. https://doi.org/10.1002/jclp.23348

Giesen-Bloo, J., van Dyck, R., Spinhoven, P., van Tilburg, W., Dirksen, C., van Asselt, T., Kremers, I., Nadort, M., & Arntz, A. (2006). Outpatient psychotherapy for borderline personality disorder: Randomized trial of schema-focused therapy vs transference-focused psychotherapy. *Archives of General Psychiatry, 63*(6), 649–658. https://doi.org/10.1001/archpsyc.63.6.649

Grant, B. F., Hasin, D. S., Stinson, F. S., Dawson, D. A., Chou, S. P., Ruan, W. J., & Pickering, R. P. (2004). Prevalence, correlates, and disability of personality disorders in the United States: Results from the National Epidemiologic Survey on Alcohol and Related Conditions. *The Journal of Clinical Psychiatry, 65*(7), 948–958. https://doi.org/10.4088/JCP.v65n0711

Grenyer, B. F. S., Lewis, K. L., Fanaian, M., & Kotze, B. (2018). Treatment of personality disorder using a whole of service stepped care approach: A cluster randomized controlled trial. *PLoS One, 13*(11), e0206472. https://doi.org/10.1371/journal.pone.0206472

Gross, J. J. (2014). Emotion regulation: Conceptual and empirical foundations. In J. J. Koenig (Ed.), *Handbook of emotion regulation* (pp. 3–20). Guilford Press.

Guilé, J. M., Boissel, L., Alaux-Cantin, S., & Garny de La Rivière, S. (2018). Borderline personality disorder in adolescents: Prevalence, diagnosis, and treatment strategies. *Adolescent Health, Medicine and Therapeutics, 9*, 199–210. https://doi.org/10.2147/AHMT.S156565

Gunderson, J. G., Bender, D., Sanislow, C., Yen, S., Rettew, J. B., Dolan-Sewell, R., Dyck, I., Morey, L. C., McGlashan, T. H., Shea, M. T., & Skodol, A. E. (2003). Plausibility and possible determinants of sudden "remissions" in borderline patients. *Psychiatry, 66*(2), 111–119. https://doi.org/10.1521/psyc.66.2.111.20614

Gunderson, J. G., & Links, P. R. (2014). *Handbook of good psychiatric management for borderline personality disorder*. American Psychiatric Publishing.

Gunderson, J. G., Morey, L. C., Stout, R. L., Skodol, A. E., Shea, M. T., McGlashan, T. H., Zanarini, M. C., Grilo, C. M., Sanislow, C. A., Yen, S., Daversa, M. T., & Bender, D. S. (2004). Major depressive disorder and borderline personality disorder revisited: Longitudinal interactions. *The Journal of Clinical Psychiatry*, *65*(8), 1049–1056. https://doi.org/10.4088/JCP.v65n0804

Gunderson, J. G., & Phillips, K. A. (1991). A current view of the interface between borderline personality disorder and depression. *The American Journal of Psychiatry*, *148*(8), 967–975. https://doi.org/10.1176/ajp.148.8.967

Gunderson, J. G., & Singer, M. T. (1975). Defining borderline patients: An overview. *The American Journal of Psychiatry*, *132*(1), 1–10. https://doi.org/10.1176/ajp.132.1.1

Gunderson, J. G., Stout, R. L., McGlashan, T. H., Shea, M. T., Morey, L. C., Grilo, C. M., Zanarini, M. C., Yen, S., Markowitz, J. C., Sanislow, C., Ansell, E., Pinto, A., & Skodol, A. E. (2011). Ten-year course of borderline personality disorder: Psychopathology and function from the Collaborative Longitudinal Personality Disorders Study. *Archives of General Psychiatry*, *68*(8), 827–837. https://doi.org/10.1001/archgenpsychiatry.2011.37

Gunderson, J. G., Stout, R. L., Shea, M. T., Grilo, C. M., Markowitz, J. C., Morey, L. C., Sanislow, C., Yen, S., Zanarini, M. C., Keuroghlian, A. S., McGlashan, T. H., & Skodol, A. E. (2014). Interactions of borderline personality disorder and mood disorders over 10 years. *The Journal of Clinical Psychiatry*, *75*(8), 829–834. https://doi.org/10.4088/JCP.13m08972

Gutheil, T. G. (1992). Suicide and suit: Liability after self-destruction. In D. Jacobs (Ed.), *Suicide and clinical practice* (pp. 147–167). American Psychiatric Publishing.

Gutheil, T. G. (2004). Suicide, suicide litigation, and borderline personality disorder. *Journal of Personality Disorders*, *18*(3), 248–256. https://doi.org/10.1521/pedi.18.3.248.35448

Haeffel, G. J., Jeronimus, B. F., Kaiser, B. N., Weaver, L. J., Soyster, P. D., Fisher, A. J., Vargas, I., Goodson, J. T., & Lu, W. (2022). Folk classification and factor rotations: Whales, sharks, and the problems with the Hierarchical Taxonomy of Psychopathology (HiTOP). *Clinical Psychological Science*, *10*(2), 259–278. https://doi.org/10.1177/21677026211002500

Haglund, A., Lysell, H., Larsson, H., Lichtenstein, P., & Runeson, B. (2019). Suicide immediately after discharge from psychiatric inpatient care: A cohort study of nearly 2.9 million discharges. *Journal of Clinical Psychiatry*, *80*(2), 18m12172. https://doi.org/10.4088/JCP.18m12172

Handelman, K., & Sumiya, F. (2022). Tolerance to stimulant medication for attention deficit hyperactivity disorder: Literature review and case report. *Brain Sciences*, *12*(8), 959. https://doi.org/10.3390/brainsci12080959

Hawn, S. E., Overstreet, C., Stewart, K. E., & Amstadter, A. B. (2015). Recent advances in the genetics of emotion regulation: A review. *Current Opinion in Psychology*, *3*, 108–116. https://doi.org/10.1016/j.copsyc.2014.12.014

Hawton, K., Zahl, D., & Weatherall, R. (2003). Suicide following deliberate self-harm: Long-term follow-up of patients who presented to a general hospital.

*The British Journal of Psychiatry, 182*(6), 537–542. https://doi.org/10.1192/bjp.182.6.537

Hechtman, L. (Ed.). (2016). *Attention deficit hyperactivity disorder: Adult outcome and its predictors.* Oxford University Press. https://doi.org/10.1093/med/9780190213589.001.0001

Herpertz, S. C., & Bertsch, K. (2022). Neuroscience and personality disorders. In S. K. Huprich (Ed.), *Personality disorders and pathology: Integrating clinical assessment and practice in the* DSM-5 *and* ICD-11 *era* (pp. 323–349). American Psychological Association. https://doi.org/10.1037/0000310-015

Herpertz, S. C., Huprich, S. K., Bohus, M., Chanen, A., Goodman, M., Mehlum, L., Moran, P., Newton-Howes, G., Scott, L., & Sharp, C. (2017). The challenge of transforming the diagnostic system of personality disorders. *Journal of Personality Disorders, 31*(5), 577–589. https://doi.org/10.1521/pedi_2017_31_338

Herzog, P., Feldmann, M., Voderholzer, U., Gärtner, T., Armbrust, M., Rauh, E., Doerr, R., Rief, W., & Brakemeier, E. L. (2020). Drawing the borderline: Predicting treatment outcomes in patients with borderline personality disorder. *Behaviour Research and Therapy, 133*, 103692. https://doi.org/10.1016/j.brat.2020.103692

Hopwood, C. J., Kotov, R., Krueger, R. F., Watson, D., Widiger, T. A., Althoff, R. R., Ansel, E. B., Bach, B., Bagby, R. M., Blais, M. A., Bornovalova, M. A., Chmielewski, M., Cicero, D. C., Conway, C., De Clercq, B., De Fruyt, F., Docherty, A. R., Eaton, N. R., Edens, J. F., . . . Zimmermann, J. (2018). The time has come for dimensional personality disorder diagnosis. *Personality and Mental Health, 12*(1), 82–86. https://doi.org/10.1002/pmh.1408

Hopwood, C. J., Mulay, A., & Waugh, M. (Eds.). (2019). *The* DSM-5 *alternative model for personality disorders: Integrating multiple paradigms of personality assessment.* Routledge. https://doi.org/10.4324/9781315205076

Horwitz, A. V., & Wakefield, J. C. (2007). *The loss of sadness: How psychiatry transformed normal sorrow into depressive disorder.* Oxford University Press. https://doi.org/10.1093/oso/9780195313048.001.0001

Iliakis, E. A., Ilagan, G. S., & Choi-Kain, L. W. (2021). Dropout rates from psychotherapy trials for borderline personality disorder: A meta-analysis. *Personality Disorders: Theory, Research, and Treatment, 12*(3), 193–206. https://doi.org/10.1037/per0000453

Iliakis, E. A., Sonley, A. K. I., Ilagan, G. S., & Choi-Kain, L. W. (2019). Treatment of borderline personality disorder: Is supply adequate to meet public health needs? *Psychiatric Services, 70*(9), 772–781. https://doi.org/10.1176/appi.ps.201900073

Jang, K. L. (2005). *The behavioral genetics of psychopathology: A clinical guide.* Routledge. https://doi.org/10.4324/9781410612724

Jang, K. L., Livesley, W. J., Vernon, P. A., & Jackson, D. N. (1996). Heritability of personality disorder traits: A twin study. *Acta Psychiatrica Scandinavica, 94*(6), 438–444. https://doi.org/10.1111/j.1600-0447.1996.tb09887.x

Janiri, D., Doucet, G. E., Pompili, M., Sani, G., Luna, B., Brent, D. A., & Frangou, S. (2020). Risk and protective factors for childhood suicidality: A US population-based study. *The Lancet Psychiatry, 7*(4), 317–326. https://doi.org/10.1016/ S2215-0366(20)30049-3

Jarvi, S., Jackson, B., Swenson, L., & Crawford, H. (2013). The impact of social contagion on non-suicidal self-injury: A review of the literature. *Archives of Suicide Research, 17*(1), 1–19. https://doi.org/10.1080/13811118.2013.748404

Jørgensen, C. R., Freund, C., Bøye, R., Jordet, H., Andersen, D., & Kjølbye, M. (2013). Outcome of mentalization-based and supportive psychotherapy in patients with borderline personality disorder: A randomized trial. *Acta Psychiatrica Scandinavica, 127*(4), 305–317. https://doi.org/10.1111/j.1600-0447.2012.01923.x

Juul, S., Jakobsen, J. C., Hestbaek, E., Jørgensen, C. K., Olsen, M. H., Rishede, M., Frandsen, F. W., Bo, S., Lunn, S., Poulsen, S., Sørensen, P., Bateman, A., & Simonsen, S. (2023). Short-term versus long-term mentalization-based therapy for borderline personality disorder: A randomized clinical trial (MBT-RCT). *Psychotherapy and Psychosomatics, 92*(5), 329–339. https://doi.org/10.1159/ 000534289

Juul, S., Jakobsen, J. C., Jørgensen, C. K., Poulsen, S., Sørensen, P., & Simonsen, S. (2023). The difference between shorter- versus longer-term psychotherapy for adult mental health disorders: A systematic review with meta-analysis. *BMC Psychiatry, 23*(1), 438. https://doi.org/10.1186/s12888-023-04895-6

Kaess, M., Brunner, R., & Chanen, A. (2014). Borderline personality disorder in adolescence. *Pediatrics, 134*(4), 782–793. https://doi.org/10.1542/peds. 2013-3677

Kazda, L., Bell, K., Thomas, R., McGeechan, K., Sims, R., & Barratt, A. (2021). Overdiagnosis of attention-deficit/hyperactivity disorder in children and adolescents: A systematic scoping review. *JAMA Network Open, 4*(4), e215335. https://doi.org/10.1001/jamanetworkopen.2021.5335

Kessler, R. C., Berglund, P., Borges, G., Nock, M., & Wang, P. S. (2005). Trends in suicide ideation, plans, gestures, and attempts in the United States, 1990–1992 to 2001–2003. *JAMA, 293*(20), 2487–2495. https://doi.org/10.1001/jama. 293.20.2487

Kessler, R. C., Chiu, W. T., Demler, O., Merikangas, K. R., & Walters, E. E. (2005). Prevalence, severity, and comorbidity of 12-month *DSM-IV* disorders in the National Comorbidity Survey Replication. *Archives of General Psychiatry, 62*(6), 617–627. https://doi.org/10.1001/archpsyc.62.6.617

Kessler, R. C., McGonagle, K. A., Zhao, S., Nelson, C. B., Hughes, M., Eshleman, S., Wittchen, H. U., & Kendler, K. S. (1994). Lifetime and 12-month prevalence of *DSM-III-R* psychiatric disorders in the United States: Results from the National Comorbidity Survey. *Archives of General Psychiatry, 51*(1), 8–19. https://doi.org/10.1001/archpsyc.1994.03950010008002

Keuroghlian, A. S., Gunderson, J. G., Pagano, M. E., Markowitz, J. C., Ansell, E. B., Shea, M. T., Morey, L. C., Sanislow, C., Grilo, C. M., Stout, R. L., Zanarini,

M. C., McGlashan, T. H., & Skodol, A. E. (2015). Interactions of borderline personality disorder and anxiety disorders over 10 years. *The Journal of Clinical Psychiatry, 76*(11), 1529–1534. https://doi.org/10.4088/JCP.14m09748

Kitayama, S., Berg, M. K., & Chopik, W. J. (2020). Culture and well-being in late adulthood: Theory and evidence. *American Psychologist, 75*(4), 567–576. https://doi.org/10.1037/amp0000614

Koenigsberg, H. W. (2010). Affective instability: Toward an integration of neuroscience and psychological perspectives. *Journal of Personality Disorders, 24*(1), 60–82. https://doi.org/10.1521/pedi.2010.24.1.60

Kothgassner, O. D., Goreis, A., Robinson, K., Huscsava, M. M., Schmahl, C., & Plener, P. L. (2021). Efficacy of dialectical behavior therapy for adolescent self-harm and suicidal ideation: A systematic review and meta-analysis. *Psychological Medicine, 51*(7), 1057–1067. https://doi.org/10.1017/S0033291721001355

Kotov, R., Krueger, R. F., Watson, D., Achenbach, T. M., Althoff, R. R., Bagby, R. M., Brown, T. A., Carpenter, W. T., Caspi, A., Clark, L. A., Eaton, N. R., Forbes, M. K., Forbush, K. T., Goldberg, D., Hasin, D., Hyman, S. E., Ivanova, M. Y., Lynam, D. R., Markon, K., . . . Zimmerman, M. (2017). The Hierarchical Taxonomy of Psychopathology (HiTOP): A dimensional alternative to traditional nosologies. *Journal of Abnormal Psychology, 126*(4), 454–477. https://doi.org/10.1037/abn0000258

Kramer, U., Grandjean, L., Beuchat, H., Kolly, S., Conus, P., de Roten, Y., Draganski, B., & Despland, J. N. (2020). Mechanisms of change in brief treatments for borderline personality disorder: A protocol of a randomized controlled trial. *Trials, 21*(1), 335. https://doi.org/10.1186/s13063-020-4229-z

Kramer, U., Kolly, S., Charbon, P., Ilagan, G. S., & Choi-Kain, L. W. (2022). Brief psychiatric treatment for borderline personality disorder as a first step of care: Adapting general psychiatric management to a 10-session intervention. *Personality Disorders: Theory, Research, and Treatment, 13*(5), 516–526. https://doi.org/10.1037/per0000511

Krantz, D. S., Shank, L. M., & Goodie, J. L. (2022). Post-traumatic stress disorder (PTSD) as a systemic disorder: Pathways to cardiovascular disease. *Health Psychology, 41*(10), 651–662. https://doi.org/10.1037/hea0001127

Krause-Utz, A., Niedtfeld, I., Knauber, J., & Schmahl, C. (2017). Neurobiology of borderline personality disorder. In B. Stanley & A. New (Eds.), *Borderline personality disorder* (pp. 83–110). Oxford University Press.

Krueger, R. F., Kotov, R., Watson, D., Forbes, M. K., Eaton, N. R., Ruggero, C. J., Simms, L. J., Widiger, T. A., Achenbach, T. M., Bach, B., Bagby, R. M., Bornovalova, M. A., Carpenter, W. T., Chmielewski, M., Cicero, D. C., Clark, L. A., Conway, C., DeClercq, B., DeYoung, C. G., . . . Zimmermann, J. (2018). Progress in achieving quan titative classification of psychopathology. *World Psychiatry, 17*(3), 282–293. https://doi.org/10.1002/wps.20566

Laporte, L., Paris, J., Bergevin, T., Fraser, R., & Cardin, J. F. (2018). Clinical outcomes of stepped care for the treatment of borderline personality disorder. *Personality and Mental Health, 12*(3), 252–264. https://doi.org/10.1002/pmh.1421

Laporte, L., Paris, J., Guttman, H., & Russell, J. (2011). Psychopathology, trauma, and personality traits in patients with borderline personality disorder and their sisters. *Journal of Personality Disorders, 25*(4), 448–462. https://doi.org/10.1521/pedi.2011.25.4.448

Lazar, S. G. (Ed.). (2010). *Psychotherapy is worth it: A comprehensive review of its cost-effectiveness.* American Psychiatric Publishing.

Lazar, S. G., Bendat, M., Gabbard, G., Levy, K., McWilliams, N., Plakun, E. M., Shedler, J., & Yeomans, F. (2018). Clinical necessity guidelines for psychotherapy, insurance medical necessity and utilization review protocols, and mental health parity. *Journal of Psychiatric Practice, 24*(3), 179–193. https://doi.org/10.1097/PRA.0000000000000309

Lazarus, S. A., Beeney, J. E., Howard, K. P., Strunk, D. R., Pilkonis, P., & Cheavens, J. S. (2020). Characterization of relationship instability in women with borderline personality disorder: A social network analysis. *Personality Disorders: Theory, Research, and Treatment, 11*(5), 312–320. https://doi.org/10.1037/per0000380

Leichsenring, F., Fonagy, P., Heim, N., Kernberg, O. F., Leweke, F., Luyten, P., Salzer, S., Spitzer, C., & Steinert, C. (2024). Borderline personality disorder: A comprehensive review of diagnosis and clinical presentation, etiology, treatment, and current controversies. *World Psychiatry, 23*(1), 4–25. https://doi.org/10.1002/wps.21156

Leichsenring, F., Heim, N., Leweke, F., Spitzer, C., Steinert, C., & Kernberg, O. F. (2023). Borderline personality disorder: A review. *JAMA, 329*(8), 670–679. https://doi.org/10.1001/jama.2023.0589

Lenzenweger, M. F., Lane, M. C., Loranger, A. W., & Kessler, R. C. (2007). DSM-IV personality disorders in the National Comorbidity Survey Replication. *Biological Psychiatry, 62*(6), 553–564. https://doi.org/10.1016/j.biopsych.2006.09.019

Linehan, M. M. (1993). *Cognitive behavior therapy for borderline personality disorder.* Guilford Press.

Linehan, M. M. (2014a). *DBT skills training handouts and worksheets* (2nd ed.). Guilford Press.

Linehan, M. M. (2014b). *DBT skills training manual* (2nd ed.). Guilford Press.

Linehan, M. M., Armstrong, H. E., Suarez, A., Allmon, D., & Heard, H. L. (1991). Cognitive–behavioral treatment of chronically parasuicidal borderline patients. *Archives of General Psychiatry, 48*(12), 1060–1064. https://doi.org/10.1001/archpsyc.1991.01810360024003

Linehan, M. M., Heard, H. L., & Armstrong, H. E. (1993). Naturalistic follow-up of a behavioral treatment for chronically parasuicidal borderline patients. *Archives of General Psychiatry, 50*(12), 971–974. https://doi.org/10.1001/archpsyc.1993.01820240055007

Livesley, W. J. (2012). Integrated treatment: A conceptual framework for an evidence-based approach to the treatment of personality disorder. *Journal of Personality Disorders, 26*(1), 17–42. https://doi.org/10.1521/pedi.2012.26.1.17

Livesley, W. J. (2017). *Integrated modular treatment for borderline personality disorder.* Cambridge University Press. https://doi.org/10.1017/9781107298613

Malone, K. M., Oquendo, M. A., Haas, G. L., Ellis, S. P., Li, S., & Mann, J. J. (2000). Protective factors against suicidal acts in major depression: Reasons for living. *The American Journal of Psychiatry, 157*(7), 1084–1088. https://doi.org/10.1176/appi.ajp.157.7.1084

Maltsberger, J. T. (1994a). Calculated risk taking in the treatment of suicidal patients: Ethical and legal problems. *Death Studies, 18*(5), 439–452. https://doi.org/10.1080/07481189408252691

Maltsberger, J. T. (1994b). Calculated risks in the treatment of intractably suicidal patients. *Psychiatry, 57*(3), 199–212. https://doi.org/10.1080/00332747.1994.11024685

May, T., Pilkington, P. D., Younan, R., & Williams, K. (2021). Overlap of autism spectrum disorder and borderline personality disorder: A systematic review and meta-analysis. *Autism Research, 14*(12), 2688–2710. https://doi.org/10.1002/aur.2619

McGirr, A., Paris, J., Lesage, A., Renaud, J., & Turecki, G. (2007). Risk factors for suicide completion in borderline personality disorder: A case-control study of cluster B comorbidity and impulsive aggression. *The Journal of Clinical Psychiatry, 68*(5), 721–729. https://doi.org/10.4088/JCP.v68n0509

McGlashan, T. H. (1986). The Chestnut Lodge follow-up study: III. Long-term outcome of borderline personalities. *Archives of General Psychiatry, 43*(1), 20–30. https://doi.org/10.1001/archpsyc.1986.01800010022003

McMain, S. F., Chapman, A. L., Kuo, J. R., Dixon-Gordon, K. L., Guimond, T. H., Labrish, C., Isaranuwatchai, I., & Streiner, D. L. (2022). The effectiveness of 6 versus 12 months of dialectical behavior therapy for borderline personality disorder: A noninferiority randomized clinical trial. *Psychotherapy and Psychosomatics, 91*(6), 382–397. https://doi.org/10.1159/000525102

McMain, S. F., Guimond, T., Barnhart, R., Habinski, L., & Streiner, D. L. (2017). A randomized trial of brief dialectical behaviour therapy skills training in suicidal patients suffering from borderline disorder. *Acta Psychiatrica Scandinavica, 135*(2), 138–148. https://doi.org/10.1111/acps.12664

McMain, S. F., Guimond, T., Streiner, D. L., Cardish, R. J., & Links, P. S. (2012). Dialectical behavior therapy compared with general psychiatric management for borderline personality disorder: Clinical outcomes and functioning over a 2-year follow-up. *The American Journal of Psychiatry, 169*(6), 650–661. https://doi.org/10.1176/appi.ajp.2012.11091416

McMain, S. F., Links, P. S., Gnam, W. H., Guimond, T., Cardish, R. J., Korman, L., & Streiner, D. L. (2009). A randomized trial of dialectical behavior therapy versus general psychiatric management for borderline personality disorder. *The American Journal of Psychiatry, 166*(12), 1365–1374. https://doi.org/10.1176/appi.ajp.2009.09010039

McNally, R. J., Robinaugh, D. J., Wu, G. W., Wang, L., Deserno, M. K., & Borsboom, D. (2015). Mental disorders as causal systems: A network approach to posttraumatic stress disorder. *Clinical Psychological Science, 3*(6), 836–849. https://doi.org/10.1177/2167702614553230

Meerwijk, E. L., Parekh, A., Oquendo, M. A., Allen, I. E., Franck, L. S., & Lee, K. A. (2016). Direct versus indirect psychosocial and behavioural interventions to prevent suicide and suicide attempts: A systematic review and meta-analysis. *The Lancet Psychiatry, 3*(6), 544–554. https://doi.org/10.1016/S2215-0366 (16)00064-X

Meuldijk, D., McCarthy, A., Bourke, M. E., & Grenyer, B. F. (2017). The value of psychological treatment for borderline personality disorder: Systematic review and cost offset analysis of economic evaluations. *PLoS One, 12*(3), e0171592. https://doi.org/10.1371/journal.pone.0171592

Mitchell, K. J. (2020). *Innate: How the wiring of our brains shapes who we are.* Princeton University Press.

Moffitt, T. E., Houts, R., Asherson, P., Belsky, D. W., Corcoran, D. L., Hammerle, M., Harrington, H., Hogan, S., Meier, M. H., Polanczyk, G. V., Poulton, R., Ramrakha, S., Sugden, K., Williams, B., Rohde, L. A., & Caspi, A. (2015). Is adult ADHD a childhood-onset neurodevelopmental disorder? Evidence from a four-decade longitudinal cohort study. *The American Journal of Psychiatry, 172*(10), 967–977. https://doi.org/10.1176/appi.ajp.2015.14101266

Moitra, M., Santomauro, D., Degenhardt, L., Collins, P. Y., Whiteford, H., Vos, T., & Ferrari, A. (2021). Estimating the risk of suicide associated with mental disorders: A systematic review and meta-regression analysis. *Journal of Psychiatric Research, 137*, 242–249. https://doi.org/10.1016/j.jpsychires.2021.02.053

Moncrieff, J., Cooper, R. E., Stockmann, T., Amendola, S., Hengartner, M. P., & Horowitz, M. A. (2023). The serotonin theory of depression: A systematic umbrella review of the evidence. *Molecular Psychiatry, 28*, 3243–3256. https://doi.org/10.1038/s41380-022-01661-0

Moran, P., Coffey, C., Romaniuk, H., Olsson, C., Borschmann, R., Carlin, J. B., & Patton, G. C. (2012). The natural history of self-harm from adolescence to young adulthood: A population-based cohort study. *The Lancet, 379*(9812), 236–243. https://doi.org/10.1016/S0140-6736(11)61141-0

Newton-Howes, G., Tyrer, P., & Johnson, T. (2006). Personality disorder and the outcome of depression: Meta-analysis of published studies. *The British Journal of Psychiatry, 188*(1), 13–20. https://doi.org/10.1192/bjp.188.1.13

Nicolini, M. E., Kim, S. Y. H., Churchill, M. E., & Gastmans, C. (2020). Should euthanasia and assisted suicide for psychiatric disorders be permitted? A systematic review of reasons. *Psychological Medicine, 50*(8), 1241–1256. https://doi.org/10.1017/S0033291720001543

Niedtfeld, I., & Bohus, M. (2019). Understanding the bio in the biosocial theory of BPD. In M. Swales (Ed.), *The Oxford handbook of dialectical behavior therapy* (pp. 23–45). Oxford University Press.

Nock, M. K. (2010). Self-injury. *Annual Review of Clinical Psychology, 6*(1), 339–363. https://doi.org/10.1146/annurev.clinpsy.121208.131258

Norcross, J. C., & Goldfried, M. R. (Eds.). (2019). *Handbook of psychotherapy integration* (3rd ed.). Oxford University Press.

Norman, R. E., Byambaa, M., De, R., Butchart, A., Scott, J., & Vos, T. (2012). The long-term health consequences of child physical abuse, emotional abuse, and neglect: A systematic review and meta-analysis. *PLoS Medicine, 9*(11), e1001349. https://doi.org/10.1371/journal.pmed.1001349

O'Connor, R. C., & Pirkis, J. (Eds.). (2016). *The international handbook of suicide prevention* (2nd ed.). Wiley. https://doi.org/10.1002/9781118903223

Olfson, M., Blanco, C., Wang, S., & Greenhill, L. L. (2013). Trends in office-based treatment of adults with stimulants in the United States. *The Journal of Clinical Psychiatry, 74*(1), 43–50. https://doi.org/10.4088/JCP.12m07975

Oliver, B. R., Trzaskowski, M., & Plomin, R. (2014). Genetics of parenting: The power of the dark side. *Developmental Psychology, 50*(4), 1233–1240. https://doi.org/10.1037/a0035388

Owens, D., Horrocks, J., & House, A. (2002). Fatal and non-fatal repetition of self-harm: Systematic review. *The British Journal of Psychiatry, 181*(3), 193–199. https://doi.org/10.1192/bjp.181.3.193

Pagura, J., Stein, M. B., Bolton, J. M., Cox, B. J., Grant, B., & Sareen, J. (2010). Comorbidity of borderline personality disorder and posttraumatic stress disorder in the U.S. population. *Journal of Psychiatric Research, 44*(16), 1190–1198. https://doi.org/10.1016/j.jpsychires.2010.04.016

Paris, J. (2003). *Personality disorders over time: Precursors, course, and outcome.* American Psychiatric Publishing.

Paris, J. (2004). Borderline or bipolar? Distinguishing borderline personality disorder from bipolar spectrum disorders. *Harvard Review of Psychiatry, 12*(3), 140–145. https://doi.org/10.1080/10673220490472373

Paris, J. (2013). Stepped care: An alternative to routine extended treatment for patients with borderline personality disorder. *Psychiatric Services, 64*(10), 1035–1037. https://doi.org/10.1176/appi.ps.201200451

Paris, J. (2015). *A concise guide to personality disorders.* American Psychological Association. https://doi.org/10.1037/14642-000

Paris, J. (2017). *Stepped care for borderline personality disorder: Making treatment brief, effective, and accessible.* Academic Press.

Paris, J. (2020a). *Overdiagnosis in psychiatry* (2nd ed.). Oxford University Press.

Paris, J. (2020b). *Social factors in the personality disorders* (2nd ed.). Cambridge University Press.

Paris, J. (2020c). *Treatment of borderline personality disorder: A guide to evidence-based practice* (2nd ed.). Guilford Press.

Paris, J. (2022a). *Nature and nurture in personality and psychopathology: A guide for clinicians.* Routledge.

Paris, J. (2022b). *Nature and nurture in psychiatry: A gene–environment model* (2nd ed.). American Psychiatric Publishing.

Paris, J. (2023a). Complex posttraumatic stress disorder and a biopsychosocial model of borderline personality disorder. *The Journal of Nervous and Mental Disease, 211*(11), 805–810. https://doi.org/10.1097/NMD.0000000000001722

Paris, J. (2023b). *Half in love with death: Managing the chronically suicidal patient* (2nd ed.). Routledge.

Paris, J. (2023c). *Myths of trauma*. Oxford University Press.

Paris, J., Bhat, V., & Thombs, B. (2015). Is adult ADHD being overdiagnosed? *The Canadian Journal of Psychiatry, 60*(7), 324–328. https://doi.org/10.1177/070674371506000705

Paris, J., & Black, D. W. (2015). Borderline personality disorder and bipolar disorder: What is the difference and why does it matter? *The Journal of Nervous and Mental Disease, 203*(1), 3–7. https://doi.org/10.1097/NMD.0000000000000225

Paris, J., & Kirmayer, L. (2016). The NIMH research domain criteria: A bridge too far. *The Journal of Nervous and Mental Disease, 24*(1), 26–32. https://doi.org/10.1097/NMD.0000000000000435

Paris, J., & Lis, E. (2013). Can sociocultural and historical mechanisms influence the development of borderline personality disorder? *Transcultural Psychiatry, 50*(1), 140–151. https://doi.org/10.1177/1363461512468105

Paris, J., & Zweig-Frank, H. (2001). A 27-year follow-up of patients with borderline personality disorder. *Comprehensive Psychiatry, 42*(6), 482–487. https://doi.org/10.1053/comp.2001.26271

Paris, J., Zweig-Frank, H., & Guzder, J. (1994a). Psychological risk factors for borderline personality disorder in female patients. *Comprehensive Psychiatry, 35*(4), 301–305. https://doi.org/10.1016/0010-440X(94)90023-X

Paris, J., Zweig-Frank, H., & Guzder, J. (1994b). Risk factors for borderline personality in male outpatients. *Journal of Nervous and Mental Disease, 182*(7), 375–380. https://doi.org/10.1097/00005053-199407000-00002

Plakun, E. M., & Villela, R. M. (2019). Psychotherapy in psychiatry: Fighting alternative facts. *Journal of Psychiatric Practice, 25*(6), 466–469. https://doi.org/10.1097/PRA.0000000000000422

Pompili, M., Girardi, P., Ruberto, A., & Tatarelli, R. (2005). Suicide in borderline personality disorder: A meta-analysis. *Nordic Journal of Psychiatry, 59*(5), 319–324. https://doi.org/10.1080/08039480500320025

Porr, V. (2010). *Overcoming borderline personality disorder*. Oxford University Press.

Porter, C., Palmier-Claus, J., Branitsky, A., Mansell, W., Warwick, H., & Varese, F. (2020). Childhood adversity and borderline personality disorder: A meta-analysis. *Acta Psychiatrica Scandinavica, 141*(1), 6–20. https://doi.org/10.1111/acps.13118

Poudel, A., Lamichhane, A., Magar, K. R., & Khanal, G. P. (2022). Non suicidal self injury and suicidal behavior among adolescents: Co-occurrence and associated risk factors. *BMC Psychiatry, 22*(1), 96. https://doi.org/10.1186/s12888-022-03763-z

Rapoport, J. L., Buchsbaum, M. S., Zahn, T. P., Weingartner, H., Ludlow, C., & Mikkelsen, E. J. (1978, February 3). Dextroamphetamine: Cognitive and behavioral effects in normal prepubertal boys. *Science, 199*(4328), 560–563. https://doi.org/10.1126/science.341313

Reeves, K. W., Vasconez, G., & Weiss, S. J. (2022). Characteristics of suicidal ideation: A systematic review. *Archives of Suicide Research*, *26*(4), 1736–1756. https://doi.org/10.1080/13811118.2021.2022551

Reichl, C., & Kaess, M. (2021). Self-harm in the context of borderline personality disorder. *Current Opinion in Psychology*, *37*, 139–144. https://doi.org/10.1016/j.copsyc.2020.12.007

Rufo, R. A. (2012). *Sexual predators among us.* Taylor & Francis.

Ruocco, A. C., Medaglia, J. D., Tinker, J. R., Ayaz, H., Forman, E. M., Newman, C. F., Williams, J. M., Hillary, F. G., Platek, S. M., Onaral, B., & Chute, D. L. (2010). Medial prefrontal cortex hyperactivation during social exclusion in borderline personality disorder. *Psychiatry Research: Neuroimaging*, *181*(3), 233–236. https://doi.org/10.1016/j.pscychresns.2009.12.001

Rutter, M. (2006). *Genes and behavior: Nature–nurture interplay explained.* Blackwell.

Rutter, M. (2012). Resilience as a dynamic concept. *Development and Psychopathology*, *24*(2), 335–344. https://doi.org/10.1017/S0954579412000028

Sauer-Zavala, S., Southward, M. W., Fruhbauerova, M., Semcho, S. A., Stumpp, N. E., Hood, C. O., Smith, M., Elhusseini, S., & Cravens, L. (2023). BPD Compass: A randomized controlled trial of a short-term, personality-based treatment for borderline personality disorder. *Personality Disorders: Theory, Research, and Treatment*, *14*(5), 534–544. https://doi.org/10.1037/per0000612

Schramm, A. T., Venta, A., & Sharp, C. (2013). The role of experiential avoidance in the association between borderline features and emotion regulation in adolescents. *Personality Disorders: Theory, Research, and Treatment*, *4*(2), 138–144. https://doi.org/10.1037/a0031389

Segal, Z. V., Williams, J. M. G., & Teasdale, J. D. (2002). *Mindfulness-based cognitive therapy for depression: A new approach to preventing relapse.* Guilford Press.

Setkowski, K., Palantza, C., van Ballegooijen, W., Gilissen, R., Oud, M., Cristea, I. A., Noma, H., Furukawa, T. A., Arntz, A., van Balkom, A. J. L. M., & Cuijpers, P. (2023). Which psychotherapy is most effective and acceptable in the treatment of adults with a (sub)clinical borderline personality disorder? A systematic review and network meta-analysis. *Psychological Medicine*, *53*(8), 3261–3280. https://doi.org/10.1017/S0033291723000685

Shah, R., & Zanarini, M. C. (2018). Comorbidity of borderline personality disorder: Current status and future directions. *Psychiatric Clinics of North America*, *41*(4), 583–593. https://doi.org/10.1016/j.psc.2018.07.009

Shannon, D. W., Giancarlo, A., & Toombs, E. (2023). Unbalanced: Mental illness, MAID and medico-legal principles. In J. Kotalik & D. W. Shannon (Eds.), *Medical assistance in dying (MAID) in Canada: Key multidisciplinary perspectives* (pp. 253–264). Springer.

Shneidman, E. S. (1996). *The suicidal mind.* Oxford University Press. https://doi.org/10.1093/oso/9780195103663.001.0001

Shorter, E. (1992). *From paralysis to fatigue: A history of psychosomatic illness in the modern era.* Free Press.

Silberschmidt, A., Lee, S., Zanarini, M., & Schulz, S. C. (2015). Gender differences in borderline personality disorder: Results from a multinational, clinical trial sample. *Journal of Personality Disorders, 29*(6), 828–838. https://doi.org/10.1521/pedi_2014_28_175

Skabeikyte, G., & Barkauskiene, R. (2021). A systematic review of the factors associated with the course of borderline personality disorder symptoms in adolescence. *Borderline Personality Disorder and Emotion Dysregulation, 8*(1), Article 12. https://doi.org/10.1186/s40479-021-00151-z

Skaug, E., Czajkowski, N. O., Waaktaar, T., & Torgersen, S. (2022). Childhood trauma and borderline personality disorder traits: A discordant twin study. *Journal of Psychopathology and Clinical Science, 131*(4), 365–374. https://doi.org/10.1037/abn0000755

Slotema, C. W., Blom, J. D., Niemantsverdriet, M. B. A., & Sommer, I. E. C. (2018). Auditory verbal hallucinations in borderline personality disorder and the efficacy of antipsychotics: A systematic review. *Frontiers in Psychiatry, 9*, 347. https://doi.org/10.3389/fpsyt.2018.00347

Soler, J., Pascual, J. C., Tiana, T., Cebrià, A., Barrachina, J., Campins, M. J., Gich, I., Alvarez, E., & Pérez, V. (2009). Dialectical behaviour therapy skills training compared to standard group therapy in borderline personality disorder: A 3-month randomised controlled clinical trial. *Behaviour Research and Therapy, 47*(5), 353–358. https://doi.org/10.1016/j.brat.2009.01.013

Soloff, P. H., Feske, U., & Fabio, A. (2008). Mediators of the relationship between childhood sexual abuse and suicidal behavior in borderline personality disorder. *Journal of Personality Disorders, 22*(3), 221–232. https://doi.org/10.1521/pedi.2008.22.3.221

Soloff, P. H., Lynch, K. G., & Kelly, T. M. (2002). Childhood abuse as a risk factor for suicidal behavior in borderline personality disorder. *Journal of Personality Disorders, 16*(3), 201–214. https://doi.org/10.1521/pedi.16.3.201.22542

Sonley, A., & Choi-Kain, L. (2021). *Good psychiatric management and dialectical behavior therapy.* American Psychiatric Publishing.

Spong, A. J., Clare, I. C. H., Galante, J., Crawford, M. J., & Jones, P. B. (2021). Brief psychological interventions for borderline personality disorder: A systematic review and meta-analysis of randomised controlled trials. *Clinical Psychology Review, 83*, 101937. https://doi.org/10.1016/j.cpr.2020.101937

Steck, N., Egger, M., Maessen, M., Reisch, T., & Zwahlen, M. (2013). Euthanasia and assisted suicide in selected European countries and US states: Systematic literature review. *Medical Care, 51*(10), 938–944. https://doi.org/10.1097/MLR.0b013e3182a0f427

Steiger, H., & Bruce, K. R. (2004). Personality traits and disorders associated with anorexia nervosa, bulimia nervosa, and binge eating disorder. In *Clinical handbook of eating disorders* (pp. 233–256). CRC Press.

Stepp, S. D., Lazarus, S. A., & Byrd, A. L. (2016). A systematic review of risk factors prospectively associated with borderline personality disorder: Taking stock and moving forward. *Personality Disorders: Theory, Research, and Treatment, 7*(4), 316–323. https://doi.org/10.1037/per0000186

Stepp, S. D., Whalen, D. J., Scott, L. N., Zalewski, M., Loeber, R., & Hipwell, A. E. (2014). Reciprocal effects of parenting and borderline personality disorder symptoms in adolescent girls. *Development and Psychopathology, 26*(2), 361–378. https://doi.org/10.1017/S0954579413001041

Stern, A. (1938). Psychoanalytic investigation of and therapy in the border line group of neuroses. *The Psychoanalytic Quarterly, 7*(4), 467–489. https://doi.org/10.1080/21674086.1938.11925367

Stoffers-Winterling, J. M., Storebø, O. J., Kongerslev, M. T., Faltinsen, E., Todorovac, A., Jørgensen, M. S., Sales, C. P., Callesen, H. E., Ribeiro, J. P., Völlm, B. A., Lieb, K., & Simonsen, E. (2022). Psychotherapies for borderline personality disorder: A focused systematic review and meta-analysis. *The British Journal of Psychiatry, 221*(3), 538–552. https://doi.org/10.1192/bjp.2021.204

Stoffers-Winterling, J., Storebø, O. J., & Lieb, K. (2020). Pharmacotherapy for borderline personality disorder: An update of published, unpublished and ongoing studies. *Current Psychiatry Reports, 22*(8), 37. https://doi.org/10.1007/s11920-020-01164-1

Stone, M. H. (1990). *The fate of borderline patients*. Guilford Press.

Storebø, O. J., Stoffers-Winterling, J. M., Völlm, B. A., Kongerslev, M. T., Mattivi, J. T., Jørgensen, M. S., Faltinsen, E., Todorovac, A., Sales, C. P., Callesen, H. E., Lieb, K., & Simonsen, E. (2020). Psychological therapies for people with borderline personality disorder. *Cochrane Database of Systematic Reviews*. https://doi.org/10.1002/14651858.CD012955

Stulz, N., Lutz, W., Kopta, S. M., Minami, T., & Saunders, S. M. (2013). Dose–effect relationship in routine outpatient psychotherapy: Does treatment duration matter? *Journal of Counseling Psychology, 60*(4), 593–600. https://doi.org/10.1037/a0033589

Tam, V., Patel, N., Turcotte, M., Bossé, Y., Paré, G., & Meyre, D. (2019). Benefits and limitations of genome-wide association studies. *Nature Reviews Genetics, 20*(8), 467–484. https://doi.org/10.1038/s41576-019-0127-1

Temes, C. M., Frankenburg, F. R., Fitzmaurice, G. M., & Zanarini, M. C. (2019). Deaths by suicide and other causes among patients with borderline personality disorder and personality-disordered comparison subjects over 24 years of prospective follow-up. *Journal of Clinical Psychiatry, 80*(1), 18m12436. https://doi.org/10.4088/JCP.18m12436

Temes, C. M., & Zanarini, M. C. (2018). The longitudinal course of borderline personality disorder. *Psychiatric Clinics of North America, 41*(4), 685–694. https://doi.org/10.1016/j.psc.2018.07.002

Tomko, R. L., Trull, T. J., Wood, P. K., & Sher, K. J. (2014). Characteristics of borderline personality disorder in a community sample: Comorbidity, treatment utilization, and general functioning. *Journal of Personality Disorders, 28*(5), 734–750. https://doi.org/10.1521/pedi_2012_26_093

Trull, T. J., Freeman, L. K., Vebares, T. J., Choate, A. M., Helle, A. C., & Wycoff, A. M. (2018). Borderline personality disorder and substance use disorders: An updated review. *Borderline Personality Disorder and Emotion Dysregulation, 5*(1), 15. https://doi.org/10.1186/s40479-018-0093-9

Trull, T. J., Jahng, S., Tomko, R. L., Wood, P. K., & Sher, K. J. (2010). Revised NESARC personality disorder diagnoses: Gender, prevalence, and comorbidity with substance dependence disorders. *Journal of Personality Disorders, 24*(4), 412–426. https://doi.org/10.1521/pedi.2010.24.4.412

Turkheimer, E. (2000). Three laws of behavior genetics and what they mean. *Current Directions in Psychological Science, 9*(5), 160–164. https://doi.org/10.1111/1467-8721.00084

Twenge, J. (2023). *Generations.* Simon & Schuster.

Tyrer, P., & Mulder, R. (2018). Dissecting the elements of borderline personality disorder. *Personality and Mental Health, 12*(2), 91–92. https://doi.org/10.1002/pmh.1422

Tyrer, P., & Mulder, R. (2022). *Personality disorder: From evidence to understanding.* Cambridge University Press. https://doi.org/10.1017/9781108951685

Valdivieso-Jiménez, G., Pino-Zavaleta, D. A., Campos-Rodriguez, S. K., Ortiz-Saavedra, B., Fernández, M. F., & Benites-Zapata, V. A. (2023). Efficacy and safety of aripiprazole in borderline personality disorder: A systematic review. *Psychiatric Quarterly, 94*(4), 541–557. https://doi.org/10.1007/s11126-023-10045-8

van der Kolk, B. (2015). *The body keeps the score: Brain, mind, and body in the healing of trauma.* Penguin.

Van Wel, B., Kockmann, I., Blum, N., Pfohl, B., Black, D. W., & Heesterman, W. (2006). STEPPS group treatment for borderline personality disorder in The Netherlands. *Annals of Clinical Psychiatry, 18*(1), 63–67. https://doi.org/10.1080/10401230500464760

Videler, A. C., Hutsebaut, J., Schulkens, J. E. M., Sobczak, S., & van Alphen, S. P. J. (2019). A life span perspective on borderline personality disorder. *Current Psychiatry Reports, 21*(7), Article 51. https://doi.org/10.1007/s11920-019-1040-1

Volkert, J., Gablonski, T. C., & Rabung, S. (2018). Prevalence of personality disorders in the general adult population in Western countries: Systematic review and meta-analysis. *The British Journal of Psychiatry, 213*(6), 709–715. https://doi.org/10.1192/bjp.2018.202

Vos, T., Allen, C., Arora, M., Barber, R. M., Bhutta, Z. A., Brown, A., Carter, A., Casey, D. C., Charlson, F. J., Chen, A. Z., Coggeshall, M., Cornaby, L., Dandona, L., Dicker, D. J., Dilegge, T., Erskine, H. E., Ferrari, A. J., Fitzmaurice, C., Fleming, T., . . . Murray, C. J. L. (2016). Global, regional, and national incidence, prevalence, and years lived with disability for 310 diseases and injuries, 1990–2015: A systematic analysis for the Global Burden of Disease Study 2015. *The Lancet, 388*(10053), 1545–1602. https://doi.org/10.1016/S0140-6736(16)31678-6

Wampold, B. E., & Imel, Z. E. (2015). *The great psychotherapy debate: The evidence for what makes psychotherapy work* (2nd ed.). Erlbaum. https://doi.org/10.4324/9780203582015

Weinberg, I., Ronningstam, E., Goldblatt, M. J., Schechter, M., & Maltsberger, J. T. (2011). Common factors in empirically supported treatments of borderline personality disorder. *Current Psychiatry Reports, 13*(1), 60–68. https://doi.org/10.1007/s11920-010-0167-x

Wertz, J., Caspi, A., Ambler, A., Arseneault, L., Belsky, D. W., Danese, A., Fisher, H. L., Matthews, T., Richmond-Rakerd, L. S., & Moffitt, T. E. (2020). Borderline symptoms at age 12 signal risk for poor outcomes during the transition to adulthood: Findings from a genetically sensitive longitudinal cohort study. *Journal of the American Academy of Child & Adolescent Psychiatry, 59*(10), 1165–1177.E2. https://doi.org/10.1016/j.jaac.2019.07.005

Wichers, M., Schreuder, M. J., Goekoop, R., & Groen, R. N. (2019). Can we predict the direction of sudden shifts in symptoms? Transdiagnostic implications from a complex systems perspective on psychopathology. *Psychological Medicine, 49*(3), 380–387. https://doi.org/10.1017/S0033291718002064

Widiger, T. A., & Costa, P. T., Jr. (Eds.). (2013). *Personality disorders and the five-factor model of personality* (3rd ed.). American Psychological Association. https://doi.org/10.1037/13939-000

Williams, L. (1998). A "classic" case of borderline personality disorder. *Psychiatric Services, 49*(2), 173–174. https://doi.org/10.1176/ps.49.2.173

Winsper, C. (2021). Borderline personality disorder: Course and outcomes across the lifespan. *Current Opinion in Psychology, 37*, 94–97. https://doi.org/10.1016/j.copsyc.2020.09.010

Witt, S. H., Streit, F., Jungkunz, M., Frank, J., Awasthi, S., Reinbold, C. S., Treutlein, J., Degenhardt, F., Forstner, A. J., Heilmann-Heimbach, S., Dietl, L., Schwarze, C. E., Schendel, D., Strohmaier, J., Abdellaoui, A., Adolfsson, R., Air, T. M., Akil, H., Alda, M., . . . Rietschel, M. (2017). Genome-wide association study of borderline personality disorder reveals genetic overlap with bipolar disorder, major depression and schizophrenia. *Translational Psychiatry, 7*(6), e1155. https://doi.org/10.1038/tp.2017.115

Woodbridge, J., Reis, S., Townsend, M. L., Hobby, L., & Grenyer, B. F. S. (2021). Searching in the dark: Shining a light on some predictors of non-response to psychotherapy for borderline personality disorder. *PLoS One, 16*(7), e0255055. https://doi.org/10.1371/journal.pone.0255055

World Health Organization. (2019). *International statistical classification of diseases and related health problems* (11th ed.). https://icd.who.int/en

Yeomans, F., Clarkin, J., & Kernberg, O. (2002). *A primer for transference-focused psychotherapy for borderline personality disorder.* Jason Aronson.

Young, J. E. (1999). *Cognitive therapy for personality disorders: A schema-focused approach* (3rd ed.). Professional Resource Exchange.

Yuan, Y., Lee, H., Eack, S. M., & Newhill, C. E. (2023). A systematic review of the association between early childhood trauma and borderline personality disorder. *Journal of Personality Disorders, 37*(1), 16–35. https://doi.org/10.1521/pedi.2023.37.1.16

Zanarini, M. C. (Ed.). (2005). *Borderline personality disorder.* CRC Press.

Zanarini, M. C. (2009). Psychotherapy of borderline personality disorder. *Acta Psychiatrica Scandinavica, 120*(5), 373–377. https://doi.org/10.1111/j.1600-0447.2009.01448.x

Zanarini, M. C. (2019). *In the fullness of time: Recovery from borderline personality disorder.* Oxford University Press.

Zanarini, M. C., & Frankenburg, F. R. (2008). A preliminary, randomized trial of psychoeducation for women with borderline personality disorder. *Journal of Personality Disorders, 22*(3), 284–290. https://doi.org/10.1521/pedi.2008.22.3.284

Zanarini, M. C., Gunderson, J. G., Frankenburg, F. R., & Chauncey, D. L. (1989). The revised Diagnostic Interview for Borderlines: Discriminating BPD from other Axis II disorders. *Journal of Personality Disorders, 3*(1), 10–18. https://doi.org/10.1521/pedi.1989.3.1.10

Zanarini, M. C., Reichman, C. A., Frankenburg, F. R., Reich, D. B., & Fitzmaurice, G. (2010). The course of eating disorders in patients with borderline personality disorder: A 10-year follow-up study. *International Journal of Eating Disorders, 43*(3), 226–232. https://doi.org/10.1002/eat.20689

Zimmerman, M. (2015). Borderline personality disorder: A disorder in search of advocacy. *The Journal of Nervous and Mental Disease, 203*(1), 8–12. https://doi.org/10.1097/NMD.0000000000000226

Zimmerman, M. (2016). Improving the recognition of borderline personality disorder in a bipolar world. *Journal of Personality Disorders, 30*(3), 320–335. https://doi.org/10.1521/pedi_2015_29_195

Zimmerman, M., & Morgan, T. A. (2013). The relationship between borderline personality disorder and bipolar disorder. *Dialogues in Clinical Neuroscience, 15*(2), 155–169. https://doi.org/10.31887/DCNS.2013.15.2/mzimmerman

Zimmerman, M., Rothschild, L., & Chelminski, I. (2005). The prevalence of *DSM-IV* personality disorders in psychiatric outpatients. *The American Journal of Psychiatry, 162*(10), 1911–1918. https://doi.org/10.1176/appi.ajp.162.10.1911

Zlotnick, C., Rothschild, L., & Zimmerman, M. (2002). The role of gender in the clinical presentation of patients with borderline personality disorder. *Journal of Personality Disorders, 16*(3), 277–282. https://doi.org/10.1521/pedi.16.3.277.22540

# Index

## A

Acceptance, radical, 69, 75
Access, to fatal means of suicide, 105
Access to therapy, 20, 85–97
    access to treatment, 85–87
    duration of therapy, 93–94
    efficacy, effectiveness, and cost-
        effectiveness, 94–95
    evidence for brief therapy, 87–88
    role of family support, 95–97
    stepped care, 88–92
Acute suicidality, 99–101
Addictions, 66
ADHD. *See* Attention deficit hyperactivity
    disorder
Adolescence, 8, 37–41, 71, 72, 101–102
Adult ADHD, 25–27
Adulthood, 40–44
Adversities, childhood, 57, 75
Advocacy, 95–96
Affective instability, 74
Affective symptoms, 15
Affectivity, 17
Alternative Model for Personality
    Disorders (AMPD), 16–17
Anankastia, 17
Antidepressants, 77–78
Antipsychotic drugs, 77–78
Anxiety, 21–22
Aripiprazole, 77
Attention deficit hyperactivity disorder
    (ADHD), 7, 25–27, 78
Australia, 90
Autism spectrum disorder, 27

## B

Beautrais, A. L., 104
Behavioral skills, 74
Behavior genetics, 55
Belgium, 107
Benzodiazipines, 78
Big Five personality model (FFM), 13,
    17–18
Biological factors, in BPD, 53–55
Biopsychosocial model, 47–49
Biopsychosocial risk factors, 61–62
Biopsychosocial theory, 47–62
    applying BPS model to BPD,
        51–53
    biological factors in BPD, 53–55
    biopsychosocial model, 47–49
    biopsychosocial risk factors, 61–62
    clinical implications of, 60–61
    genetics, traumatic events, and
        social stressors, 49–51
    psychological factors in BPD,
        55–58
    social risk factors in BPD, 59
Biosocial model, 54, 58
Biosocial theory-based dialectical
    behavior therapy, 57
Bipolar disorders, 22–24
Bohus, M., 54
Borderline personality disorder (BPD)
    key features of, 11–13
    as term, 5, 13–14
Brain scans, 54
Brief therapy, 66–67, 87–88

## C

Canada, 73, 86, 92, 107
CBT (cognitive behavior therapy), 21, 68
Childhood adversities, 57, 75
Childhood sexual abuse, 57
Childhood trauma, 56, 57
Clinical implications, of biopsychosocial
    theory, 60–61
Clinician's illusion, 40, 42
Clinics, extended care, 92
CLPS (Collaborative Longitudinal
    Personality Disorders Study), 40–41
Cognitive behavior therapy (CBT), 21, 68
Collaborative Longitudinal Personality
    Disorders Study (CLPS), 40–41
Commitment, to therapy, 92
Common factors model, 76
Community prevalence, 33–37
Comorbidities, 5, 12, 20–31, 90
Complex posttraumatic stress disorder
    (CPTSD), 28, 56
Compulsivity, 17
Co-occurrences, 12, 31
Cost, of therapy, 70
Cost-effectiveness, of therapy, 67, 94–95
CPTSD (complex posttraumatic stress
    disorder), 28, 56
Criticism, constant, 52
Cutting, 21, 101–102

## D

DBT. See Dialectical behavior therapy
Depression, 7, 20–22
Detachment, 17
Development, of identity, 59
Diagnosis and misdiagnosis, of BPD, 11–31
    BPD, as term, 13–14
    comorbidities and differential diagnosis,
        20–31
    and DSM system, 14–17
    and ICD-11, 17–18
    key features of BPD, 11–13
    and trait dimensions, 18–20
Diagnostic and Statistical Manual of Mental
    Disorders (DSM), 12, 14–17, 19
Dialectical behavior therapy (DBT), 7,
    57–58, 68–74, 87
Differential diagnosis, 20–31
Differential susceptibility to the
    environment, 49
Dimensional systems, 15–18

Disinhibition, 17
Dissociality, 17
Distress tolerance, 66
Double-hit, 51
Dropouts, from psychotherapy, 81
Drugs, 60, 77–79
DSM. See Diagnostic and Statistical Manual
    of Mental Disorders
Dysfunctional families, 39, 56, 58

## E

Eating disorders, 30–31, 59, 66, 90
Efficacy, of therapy, 7, 94–95
Efficacy and effectiveness, of therapy, 7,
    94–95
Emergency room visits, 86, 89, 90,
    100–101
Emotional abuse, 52, 55, 57
Emotional neglect, 6, 55, 57
Emotion dysregulation, 11, 38, 41, 54–55,
    74
Emotion regulation, 66, 87
Employment, 78–79, 90
Engel, G., 47
Environment, differential susceptibility
    to, 49
Environmental factors, 48–49
Environment-gene interactions, 51
Epidemiological surveys, 34
Equifinality, 39
ER visits. See Emergency room visits
Evidence-based therapies, 71–73

## F

Failure of validation, 52
Families, of patients, 96
Family dysfunction, 39, 56, 58
Family support, role of, 95–97
FFM (Five-factor personality model),
    13, 17–18
Firearms, 104–105
Five-factor personality model (FFM),
    13, 17–18
Frontal lobe, 54

## G

Gender differences, 36, 57, 104
General psychiatric management (GPM),
    7, 72, 76

General psychiatric management for adolescents (GPM-A), 72
Genetics, 6, 48, 49–51, 53–55
Good psychiatric management. *See* General psychiatric management
GPM. *See* General psychiatric management
GPM-A. *See* General psychiatric management for adolescents
Gunderson, J. G., 14

**H**

Hanging, 104–105
Harvard University, 96
Heritability gap, 53
Heritable traits, 48–50
Hierarchical Taxonomy of Psychopathology (HiToP), 19
Hoffmann, P., 95
Hospitalization, for suicide attempts, 100–101, 105. *See also* Emergency room visits
Hypomania, 22

**I**

*ICD-11 (International Classification of Diseases, 11th ed.)*, 17–18
Identity development, 59
Impulsive symptoms, 15
Impulsivity, 11, 38, 41–42
Insomnia, 77
Insurance, mental health, 86
*International Classification of Diseases, 11th ed. (ICD-11)*, 17–18
Internet, 101–102
Interpersonal skills, 74

**K**

Kramer, U., 87

**L**

Lack of focus, 26
Lamotrigine, 77–78
Life events, adverse, 49–50
Life spans, of BPD patients, 45
Linehan, M. M., 54, 69–70, 106
Litigation, 107–108
Livesley, W. J., 73, 76

**M**

MBT (mentalization-based treatment), 7, 71–72
McGill University, 92
McLean Hospital, 96
McLean Study of Adult Development (MSAD), 40–41
Medications, 60, 77–79
Mental health insurance, 86
Mentalization, 68
Mentalization-based treatment (MBT), 7, 71–72
Micropsychotic symptoms, 11–12, 24, 109
Misdiagnosis. *See* Diagnosis and misdiagnosis
Mood stabilizers, 77
Mood swings, 20–23
MSAD (McLean Study of Adult Development), 40–41
Multifinality, 39

**N**

Naltrexone, 78
National Comorbidity Survey, 34, 104
National Education Alliance for Borderline Personality Disorder (NEA-BPD), 95
National Institute of Mental Health (NIMH), 95, 96
Netherlands, 107
Neuroanatomical pathways, 54
Neuroscience, 48
Niedtfeld, I., 54
NIMH (National Institute of Mental Health), 95, 96
Nonsuicidal self-injury (NSSI), 21, 101–102

**O**

Outcomes, 40–44. *See also* Prevalence, precursors, and outcomes

**P**

Pagers, 74–75
Parents, of patients, 96
Personality disorders (PD), 15, 29–30, 33, 59, 66, 91
Pharmacological interventions, 60, 77–79
Pittsburgh Girls Study, 39
Placebo effects, 26

Porr, V., 95
Porter, C., 52
Posttraumatic stress disorder (PTSD), 7, 28–29, 49–50
Precursors. *See* Prevalence, precursors, and outcomes
Prediction, of suicidality, 103–105
Prevalence, precursors, and outcomes
    BPD in adulthood, and long-term outcome, 40–44
    clinical prevalence, 36–37
    outcome of suicidality, 45–46
    precursors, and adolescent onset, 37–41
    prevalence, in the community, 33–37
Prevention, of suicidality, 103–105
Psychache, 107
Psychological factors, 55–58
Psychosis, 24
Psychotherapy, 60
    dropouts, 81
    efficacy and effectiveness of, 7, 94–95
    how it helps, 73–75
    integration of, 76–77
    length of, 66–67, 70, 86, 93–94
    management of suicidality in, 105–110
    response to, 81–82
    specific and nonspecific factors in, 65–69
PTSD. *See* Posttraumatic stress disorder

**Q**

Quetiapine, 77

**R**

Radical acceptance, 69, 75
Randomized clinical trials (RCTs), 94
RDoC (Research Domain Criteria framework), 19
Recovery, 43–44, 79–81
Relationships, interpersonal, 11, 15, 79, 91
Research, future directions for, 113–114
Research Domain Criteria framework (RDoC), 19
Risk factors, biopsychosocial, 61–62
Rutter, M., 56

**S**

Schema therapy, 74. *See also* CBT (cognitive behavior therapy)

School enrollment, 36, 41, 79–80, 90–91
Selective serotonin reuptake inhibitors (SSRIs), 77
Self-harm, 21, 37–38, 51, 70
Sexual abuse, childhood, 57
Shared environmental factors, 48
Sibling studies, 52. *See also* Twin studies
Singer, M. T., 14
Social contagion, 51, 101–102
Social risk factors, in BPD, 59
Social stressors, 49–51
Societies, traditional, 59
SSRIs (selective serotonin reuptake inhibitors), 77
Steeling, 53
Stepped care, 88–92
STEPPS (Systems Training for Emotional Predictability and Problem Solving), 73, 87
Stimulants, 78
Substance use and abuse, 30–31, 59, 90
Suicides and suicidality, 99–110
    assisted suicide, 107
    attempted vs. completed, 108–109
    chronic, 99–103
    completed suicides, 109
    hospitalization for, 100–101, 105
    managing, in psychotherapy, 105–110
    NSSI (nonsuicidal self-injury), 101–102
    outcome of, 45–46
    prediction and prevention, 103–105
    suicidal ideation, 37–38, 103–105, 108
    suicide attempts, 100–101, 106, 108–110
    suicide rate, 33, 37, 104
Surveys, epidemiological, 34
Switzerland, 87, 107
Systems Training for Emotional Predictability and Problem Solving (STEPPS), 73, 87

**T**

TARA4BPD (Treatment and Research Advancements National Association for Borderline Personality Disorder), 96
Targeted therapy, 67
TAU (treatment as usual), 66

Temperament, 48
TFP. *See* Transference-focused
    psychotherapy
Therapy, duration of, 93–94. *See also*
    Access to therapy
Time-limited therapy, 67
Tolerance, of distress, 66
Traditional societies, 59
Trait dimensions, 17, 18–20
Transference-focused psychotherapy
    (TFP), 68, 72, 74
Trauma, 56
Trauma, childhood, 56–57
Traumatic events, 6, 49–51
Traumatology, 55
Treatability, 79–81
Treatment, access to, 85–87
Treatment and Research Advancements
    National Association for Borderline
    Personality Disorder (TARA4BPD), 96
Treatment as usual (TAU), 66

Treatment methods, 65–83
    DBT, 69–71
    how psychotherapy helps, 73–75
    other evidence-based therapies, 71–73
    pharmacological interventions, 77–79
    psychotherapy integration, 76–77
    response to psychotherapy, 81–82
    specific and nonspecific factors in
        psychotherapy, 65–69
    treatability and recovery, 79–81
Twin studies, 6, 37, 48, 52, 55

**U**

Unemployment, 78–79, 90
University of Montreal, 92
Unshared environmental factors, 48

**V**

Validation, failure of, 52

# About the Author

**Joel Paris, MD, PhD,** was born in New York City, but has spent most of his life in Canada. He obtained an MD from McGill University, where he also trained in psychiatry. Dr. Paris has served as department chair of the Department of Psychiatry at McGill University and is now Emeritus Professor of Psychiatry. He is a former editor-in-chief of the *Canadian Journal of Psychiatry*. His main clinical and research interest is borderline personality disorder, about which he has written more than 200 research papers, 60 book chapters, and 30 books. Dr. Paris heads personality disorder clinics at two hospitals in the McGill network.